THE DON'T SWEAT GUIDE
TO WEIGHT LOSS

D0963929

Other books by the editors of Don't Sweat Press

The Don't Sweat Affirmations
The Don't Sweat Guide for Couples
The Don't Sweat Guide for Graduates
The Don't Sweat Guide for Grandparents
The Don't Sweat Guide for Parents
The Don't Sweat Guide for Moms
The Don't Sweat Guide for Weddings
The Don't Sweat Guide to Golf
The Don't Sweat Stories
The Don't Sweat Guide to Travel
The Don't Sweat Guide to Taxes

THE DON'T SWEAT GUIDE TO WEIGHT LOSS

Feeling at Peace with Your Body

By the Editors of Don't Sweat Press
Foreword by Richard Carlson, Ph.D.

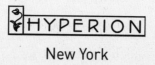

New York

Always consult your physician before beginning
any weight loss or exercise program.

Hyperion books are available for special promotions and premiums.
For details contact Hyperion Special Markets, 77 West 66th Street,
11th floor, New York, New York, 10023, or call 212-456-0100.

ISBN: 0-7868-8810-5

FIRST EDITION

10 9 8 7 6 5 4 3 2 1

Contents

Foreword

Anyone who has ever struggled with their weight knows the importance of perspective. After all, it's not easy losing weight. For most of us, including myself, there have been, or will be, a few disappointments that go along with the success. It seems to come with the territory. In order to stay on track and keep our eye on the goal, it's helpful to keep our spirits high.

Collectively, our weight is extremely important to many of us. Unfortunately, in many cases, it becomes an obsession. Somehow, we allow our own goals to interfere with our sense of well-being and enjoyment of life. We convince ourselves that we can only be content "if and when" we lose those extra pounds. We become frustrated and stressed when we step on the scale or look in the mirror.

But isn't the most important ingredient of all the way we approach our goals and the way we feel about ourselves? Wouldn't it be nice if we could enjoy, not only the end result (our desired weight), but each step along the way—the process? I think it's not only possible to approach weight loss in this light, but necessary as well. In my opinion, our greatest chance of success occurs when we are optimistic and wise; when we don't allow disappointment or the failure to meet an expectation to interfere with our sense of purpose. We are better able to stick to a plan, live with discipline, and make healthy choices, when we approach our lives—and goals—with kindness, when we have self-respect and self-love, independent of the number that shows up on the scale.

The editors of Don't Sweat Press have written an excellent book that points us in this direction. Rather than focus their attention on a specific diet, they instead help us to embrace any healthy program by encouraging us to be all we can be. Their advice helps us keep our perspective and sense of humor, while still acknowledging and working toward our ultimate goals. This book helps us become wiser and more reflective about the decisions we make, and how to stay on track without driving ourselves crazy! And, when we get off track, it helps us re-ignite our inner resiliency—the ultimate key to success.

If you are one of the millions of people who are concerned about your weight, I wish you the best of luck in achieving your goals. I know you have it in you to be as fit and healthy as your heart desires. Most importantly, however, I hope you will discover the wisdom within yourself to make yourself happy and filled with peace.

Treasure yourself, exactly as you are.

Richard Carlson
Benicia, CA, March 2002

THE DON'T SWEAT GUIDE
TO WEIGHT LOSS

1.

Understand Your Body Type

Based on the rhetoric in the many advertisements for weight-loss programs and products today, with the right help, anyone can become slim, trim, and shapely. It's an alluring goal that unfortunately sets many people up for disappointment and discouragement. While it's true that with information and discipline, most people can lose excess weight and tone muscle, it is not true that all of them will then take on the ideal proportions currently dictated by social standards. Neither is it true that each of them will achieve results with the same amount of effort.

Both scientific research and common sense tell us that bodies come in many shapes, sizes, and types. Aside from differences in height, there are variables in skeleton, digestive tract, metabolism, bone size and density, angularity, and natural body fat and muscularity. Simply interpreted, this means that there cannot possibly be a one-for-all "ideal" body. The many characteristics of body type create many ideals within the range of good health and fitness.

W. H. Sheldon developed a system for classifying body types. There is the "ectomorphic" body, which is characterized by a light build and slight muscles. The "endomorphic" body, in contrast, tends to softness, roundness, and a heavy build. Then there's the huskier, muscular "mesomorphic" body. These are general categories with many variations among them. But the essential fact remains: We start with a "type" of physique, and the best we can hope for—short of reconstructive surgery—is whatever constitutes the best for our type.

An important early step in dealing with weight loss is a recognition and acceptance of what you cannot change about your body. Just as willpower and a good diet will not add inches to your natural height, the best weight-loss program in the world will not turn a mesomorph into an ectomorph.

Take the time to know and understand your body type. Learn to appreciate it instead of struggling to make it something it is not. If you need convincing that your body is "okay," find people of similar basic build whose physical condition you admire. Build your self-image from the blueprint of your own makeup and you'll save yourself a lot of frustration and recrimination.

2.

Think Cruise, Not Crash

One of the headline makers in the land of modern weight loss is the quick drop. "Lose 30 Pounds in 30 Days," the ads offer, or, "Don't Wait for the Weight to be Gone! Shape Up for Summer in Three Easy Weeks!" Usually such come-ons tout a drug, a "system," or a diet that goes to extremes for a short period of time to get quick results. In fact, in some cases, those quick results are possible. Statistics show, however, that "easy-off" weight is almost always "easy-on" again within a year of the loss. Over time, if repeated, such quick, wide swings make weight loss increasingly difficult. In other words, the quick loss is an illusion.

As tempting as a crash program for weight loss may be, it will never offer the long-range results that come from a slow and steady approach. Taking time allows for the need to change longstanding habits—a habit is made or broken in about six weeks—that have typically subverted the desire to reach a weight goal. Taking time means that a well-balanced diet can be devised and maintained, rather than depending on a lopsided program that forces a quick loss. Taking time also makes room for a broader focus on overall good health and fitness. Substantive changes in muscle mass, body tone, and energy all have a positive effect on weight control, but they require change over time.

Give yourself your best chance at success by giving yourself time. Think in terms of "six months from now" or "this time next year" if you're aiming to lose anything more than a few pounds. Get medically sound information about the various factors that enhance weight loss and weight control, and pay attention to the risks involved in rapid loss. Forget "crash" tactics. They are about as wholesome and effective as the word implies. Instead, think "cruise," and learn to pace yourself in a way that reduces stress and increases long-term success.

3.

Don't Worry About Food

One of the sad results that can grow out of a weight-loss effort is food-focused stress. Because we know that food is a central component of weight loss and control, we can become obsessed with the subject. We spend more time and energy than necessary worrying about what we can or cannot eat, how much we just ate, when we'll get to eat again, and how to avoid eating again. We know that some foods tend to add up to body fat more quickly; we find ourselves fretting over labels and endlessly calculating fat-to-protein ratios. Sometimes, we get to a point where we can't push food out of our minds, and actually goad ourselves into eating more rather than less.

Food is a natural and necessary part of human life. It provides the nutrition and calories that we need, not only to survive, but also to thrive. Food grows in a seemingly endless array of colors, textures, flavors, and shapes. Its variety reflects a miraculous accommodation to a wide range of climates, seasons, soils, and water tables. Its cultivation provides a living for some and a great hobby for others. Its preparation by human hands demonstrates a plenitude of attitudes, traditions, and creativity.

With such a marvel in the mix of our lives, it seems a pity to turn it into anxiety. Attitude counts. Food needs to have a positive, balanced place in your thoughts, as well as your diet.

For example, any weight-loss goal is best met with a good plan in hand. Review your plan daily, whatever it is, to make impulsive food decisions a thing of the past. You won't have to fuss and fume over food, because you've already chosen what, when, and where you'll eat.

Remember, too, that food is primarily your body's fuel and resource for repair. When you find yourself preoccupied with food, ask yourself, "Have I fed my body what it needs?" If the answer is yes, give yourself a pat on the back and consciously redirect your attention.

Food offers pleasure to all of the senses while serving a vital physical need. Let it serve its purpose and add its pleasures with your approval and gratitude.

4.

Identify Depression Eating

All sorts of motivations send us to the kitchen at home or the snack bar at work when we aren't really hungry. Ironically, depression, a typical source of loss of appetite in some, is a frequent cause of overeating in others. Some researchers suggest that our desire to eat when we're blue has to do with imbalances in specific brain chemicals that affect mood and are stimulated by certain foods. Others tie depression eating to a need for comfort. Still others claim that dieting causes the depression in the first place and sets in motion a vicious cycle of food restriction, depression, and overeating.

Whatever the mechanics of it, eating to beat the blues provides at best a momentary salve, and almost always produces guilt and unhappiness in its wake. When you find yourself eating for seemingly no good reason, stop chewing long enough to identify what you're feeling. If you can identify the predominant emotion as unhappiness, you've taken an important first step toward learning new, more productive coping mechanisms.

Remember that eating when you are not hungry is a conditioned response, and as such, can be reconditioned or retrained. For example, suppose that you have discovered a pattern of depression eating. You have two important actions to put into place. One is to identify any common times, themes, or circumstances that seem to bring on the blues and make you want to eat. Perhaps you are brought low by the short daylight hours of winter. Maybe a call from one of your parents sends you into a tailspin. Maybe it's a problem at work or with a friend.

Once you've identified the cause, you can develop an alternative response to your mood. You may want to call friends or family to make contact with those that you know care about you. You may decide to turn on more warm-spectrum lights earlier in the day when winter sets in, or take time in the day to watch the sunset with a cup of tea or coffee. You may find it helpful to take a short walk, if you can, or turn on some music.

The point is that eating is rarely the best response to depression, especially when weight control is one of your issues. You can't learn new responses until you understand the old. Pay attention to those snacks that have nothing to do with physical hunger. If you're eating to cheer yourself up, reconsider. You have many other options, and some of them could have a far more lasting effect on beating the blues.

5.

Be an Individual

There is no end to the number of diet plans and programs. One person swears by the "grapefruit" diet, another eats nothing but meat. One eats no breakfast, a large lunch, and cereal for dinner. Go to any bookstore and browse the miles of shelf space given to diet and weight loss, and you'll begin to fathom just how much variety exists on the subject.

The catch is that people are just as various as the diet plans. We have different metabolisms, different taste and texture preferences, different internal "clocks," and different daily schedules. There is no one plan or program that is the magic answer for weight loss for all of us. Each of us brings a unique combination of background, makeup, and personal preference to the diet mix. Unless you recognize this fact, you may very well be condemned to serial dieting, and continue to find yourself frustrated, bored, discouraged, or doomed.

The answer is *not* to throw out all of the accumulated wisdom on the subject and settle in front of the television with a bag of chips. Rather, it is to learn about good nutrition and the mechanics of weight loss, and then to combine that information with what you know about yourself. A bagel at breakfast, a salad with protein at lunch, and a salad, vegetable, and protein at dinner (all fat-free) may win the day for you. But if you know that if you don't add some protein to that bagel, your stomach will be growling by ten in the morning, you may want to redesign the plan. If you have little love for meat, the all-meat program may not be for you. In fact, there may be no one diet that suits the unique you.

The more that you know about nutrition and the mechanics of weight control, the better off you will be when it comes to formulating a daily plan that suits your needs. You are an individual, and there is no reason to deny that you may have some special needs—either for health, aesthetic, or other reasons—that require a little informed redesigning of existing ideas. You'll know if you've chosen intelligently by the results. If your choices don't work the way that you want, you can try something different. It's a matter of process based on your individual needs.

6.

Consider the Company That You Keep

Peer pressure starts early in life, and for many of us, it never quits. This can be as true with food issues as with anything else. If we enjoy overindulging in food or drink, or if we have a love of rich cuisine, we may very well find others who feel and do the same. Finding friends with common interests is, in general, a healthy, life-affirming choice. However, when your common ground with friends is an activity that subverts your interest in losing weight and maintaining a healthy way of eating, you can find yourself with a peer-pressure problem that you thought you left behind in high school.

Changing eating habits is almost always an important factor in weight loss. It may be that the change requires that we also change habits surrounding food—when or how often we eat, the types of eateries that we frequent, and the kinds or amounts of food that we consume. If a friendship includes food habits we want to change, we face the double challenge of motivating ourselves, as well as resisting the enticements of friends. Don't let that stop you from pursuing a worthy goal in relation to your own health and well-being. Remember that challenges are the stuff of growth and character, not setups for failure.

Give your friends the opportunity to rise to the challenge with you. Let them know what you're doing and why. A true friend will support you. You may even discover that one or more of your food buddies would like to make the same sorts of changes that you're seeking. In that case, you will actually gain companionship and mutual accountability for positive change instead of temptation.

Short of that, consider taking a break from the food crowd while you're changing your habits. Alternatively, think about activities that you can encourage with friends that don't involve eating. Movies, museum tours, physical activities, concerts, book groups, and sports events are all options, provided you orchestrate them in such a way that they don't become excuses for culinary indulgences.

Remember, peer pressure can work in two directions. Rather than being the one who is led, become the leader. Think for yourself, and act in your own best interests. You may end up looking and feeling so good that your friends will want to follow you.

7.

Favor Flavor Over Fat

Although food trends have changed somewhat in recent years, the fact remains that some of the most eye-catching and enticing foods on the supermarket shelves are loaded with fat. So are many of the offerings on restaurant menus. High-fat and processed meats, butter, cheese, nuts and nut butters, cream, chips, cookies, and ice cream—these are the fat-rich offerings that call us. Unfortunately, they often also keep us from meeting the weight goals that we set. Habitually indulging in excessive amounts of dietary fat—more than twenty-five to thirty percent of daily calorie intake, according to most nutrition experts—usually leads to abnormal weight gain and obesity.

Why do we gravitate to fatty foods? It is probably because we have come to associate flavor with fat. Any meat lover will attest that it's the fine marbling of fat that makes for the most flavorful cut. Or that chicken or turkey is dry and bland without the fatty skin. A baked potato is all well and good, but it's the sour cream and bacon that load the spud with richness. The most mouth-watering desserts almost invariably include high amounts of butter and cream.

Fat contains a heavy concentration of calories even in the smallest portion. A full cup of green beans contains only thirty-five calories. A single tablespoon of butter or oil contains between 100 and 125 calories. It's easy to see how it can add up.

Understanding the significant role that flavor plays in fatty foods can help trim the fat out of our daily intake. Many low- or no-fat flavor enhancers are available. The trick is simply to identify such flavor boosters and learn how to make them work with a variety of foods. Get to know which herbs and spices appeal to you. Experiment with gourmet mustards, vinegars, and wines. Try the many varieties of wild mushrooms, sun-dried tomatoes, onions, leeks, shallots, garlic, or spicy peppers. Use small amounts of defatted broth in lieu of extra fat for sautéing; add a dash of soy sauce, Worcestershire sauce, citrus juice, or Tabasco to a vegetable dish. If you want a flavor boost from a higher-fat ingredient such as olives, avocado, nuts, cheese, or anchovies, settle for smaller amounts.

There's no end to the possibilities for flavor without fat. You're limited only by your imagination—so get to know where the fat hides. Commit yourself to trimming the fat calories, and make the adventure tasty with new sources of flavor.

8.

Balance Eating with Exercise

Weight loss and weight control have a direct relationship to the ratio of calories consumed to calories burned in your system. If you ingest more calories than your body is burning, your body will store the extra fuel as fat to be burned when needed. If you take in the same number of calories that you will need for the day, your body will maintain the status quo. You won't gain fat, and you won't lose it. If, on the other hand, you tip the balance in the direction of fueling your system with fewer calories than you burn, your body will draw on stored energy—fat—and burn it up to keep going. The number of calories that you need on a daily basis depends on gender, age, build, metabolism, and activity level.

When you are active, you burn more calories than when you are sedentary. All other factors being equal, it takes a 130-pound person approximately thirty calories to sit and watch TV for a half-hour. To do deskwork for the same duration burns twice that number. Play a rousing game of Ping-Pong, and the ante is upped to about a hundred calories. Walk two miles in that half-hour, and the calorie consumption is raised to something closer to 160. Thirty minutes of climbing stairs burns a fabulous 440 calories.

Add to this equation the information that the exercise not only burns the calories but also builds a greater rate of calorie burn in general. In other words, you get bonus calorie points as a result of the exercise.

Individuals who make activity a habitual part of their lives also frequently report that exercise diminishes their appetite and discourages overeating. One possible reason for this is that one of the cardio-respiratory benefits of exercise is a more *efficient* body. You don't need as many calories to meet your basic needs, so your system does not call for as much fuel.

Of course, not all equations are so direct or quantifiable. Many exercisers claim that the most meaningful benefit of their activity is the state of mind and spirit it produces. After a brisk walk or a lively game of tennis, they feel a noticeable lift in mood. Because so many people overeat to offset feelings of boredom, sadness, or loneliness, that mood change can offer a positive effect on weight loss, as well. With that sense of well-being, they turn less frequently to food for reasons other than actual hunger.

By all means, watch what you eat, and count calories if it helps. But keep in mind that you double your potential for success when you give as much attention to exercise as you do to diet.

9.

Uncover Habits from Childhood

There is much in the way that we live, especially when we're on "auto-pilot," that developed long before adulthood. This applies to the way that we eat and exercise just as certainly as to the way that we tie our shoes, greet our relatives, or throw a ball. Many of the food and activity habits of childhood have close emotional associations with family history.

Maybe you regularly relive a Friday night tradition of pizza and ice cream sundaes, or a nightly ritual of peanut-butter toast and hot chocolate. Perhaps you remember and recreate the thrill of a secret candy binge on vacation, or the no-holds-barred indulgences of holidays. Reliving these moments can serve as a warm, nostalgic journey into a familiar past. Just as easily, however, it can become a default behavior that keeps you from being true to your intentions.

A little self-awareness can go a long way. Think back to childhood days. What did your family consider a treat? What were the "traditional" meals and snacks? What did Mom offer when you had a disappointment or a victory? What attitudes prevailed concerning physical activity? How often did your family get out and do something energetic when the doldrums set in? As you consciously recall your past, you may develop a keener awareness of how much of it has continued into your present. The point is not to toss the old out indiscriminately, but rather to make realistic, conscious choices. If childhood habits serve your adult priorities, enjoy them to the hilt. If they get in your way, acknowledge it and look for new options.

10.

Know When to Eat

People who have done a lot of dieting or who have made a habit of eating more than their bodies need may find that their hunger mechanism no longer gives them an accurate read on what they actually require for good health and vitality. In other words, they feel hungry when they don't actually have any physical need for more food. For such people, it may take some conscious effort to get back in touch with physical needs. Consider a few suggestions.

Eat your meals at relatively consistent times, and make sure that they center on a well-rounded supply of fuel such as is suggested by the Food and Drug Administration's food guide pyramid. Your body is amazing; it will adjust to the rhythms of your intake and become an accurate meal clock if you give it a consistent schedule to adopt. If your meals are providing the nutrients that you need, you are much less likely to experience hunger pangs between meals.

When you first feel hungry between meals, have a glass of water. Sometimes, what we interpret as hunger is actually thirst, and downing eight to ten ounces of fresh water will actually offset the impression of hunger. In fact, regular doses of unsweetened, decaffeinated fluid help regulate body processes and can have a valuable effect on appetite in general. Nutrition experts suggest eight eight-ounce servings of water a day.

When between-meal hunger pangs strike, make it a habit to wait fifteen minutes before responding. It's amazing how often the feeling of hunger passes if you don't feed it immediately. This suggests that the feeling may have less to do with actual physical need than with some other kind of discomfort. You may be bored, tired, blue, or anxious. Generally speaking, it serves all of your needs more effectively to get to the bottom of the hunger response rather than simply feeding it. Over time, practicing the "wait and see" technique may retrain your appetite to send appropriate signals while helping you to better identify other sorts of needs.

When hunger doesn't desert you after a big glass of water and a fifteen-minute delay, make a point of choosing whole-food, high-energy snacks. Eat a piece of fresh fruit, some low-fat yogurt, a small portion of almonds, or a couple of whole-grain crackers with hummus. Drink another glass of water. If you're in the habit of eating high-fat, processed snacks, these whole-food options may not entice you at first. But many people have made the switch and found that unlike empty-calorie snacks, these whole foods satisfy energy needs without leading to overindulgence or cravings.

11.

Make Realistic Goals

Most of us enjoy the sense of accomplishment that comes with making a goal for ourselves and then meeting it. Our self-esteem grows. Motivation to set new goals grows. We feel empowered and successful.

When we consistently set goals that we do not reach, the reverse ensues. We feel like failures. Our confidence shrinks. We find ourselves tempted to give up, or we cease to take our goal-setting seriously.

Often, the source of trouble is not intrinsic weakness or even lack of will. It is quite simply an unrealistic view of what can be accomplished in a given period of time. It takes about six weeks to make or break a habit. If you're aiming to institute an exercise regime or a new way of eating, you need to take that time frame into account and pace yourself. Many people find that the best approach is to set mini-goals in such a case.

For example, rather than aiming to jog five miles three times a week and lift weights every other day, *starting tomorrow*, it might better serve real change to aim for that combination two months from now. (Remember to check with your doctor before beginning any exercise program.) Decide that for Weeks One and Two, you'll walk or jog two miles twice a week and lift two-pound weights twice a week. For Weeks Three and Four, jog two miles three times and lift three times. In Weeks Five and Six, increase the jogging to three miles and add pounds to your weights. And so on, until you reach the total that you've set as your goal. There's nothing wrong with charting out how you intend to build up to the total, week by week. In fact, it will help you remember what you're aiming for.

This slow and steady approach works equally well with diet changes. While instituting a radical change may seem like an effective way to make a big difference in a hurry, it rarely works over time. Rather than thinking in terms of starting a "diet" and losing five pounds a week, aim for a more conservative one or two pounds a week, while mapping out a week-by-week switch from present eating habits to the healthful, trim style of eating that you hope to achieve for a lifetime. The weight loss will add up before you know it. At the same time, you'll be working within the time frame needed to actually make and break habits. Best of all, you'll be incorporating a strategy for constructive change that can work in any part of your life. You'll discover just how much power you actually have to make the life that you want.

12.

Record Your Eating Habits

"I just don't understand it," says the wannabe trim individual. "I've cut out the potatoes, the bread, and the desserts. I feel like I do nothing but deprive myself. And I don't lose a single ounce!"

This is a common complaint among dieters, but the fact is that most of us take in more calories than we realize. Certainly, the food that you choose will have an effect on the speed of weight reduction. A diet low in fat and high in fiber and nutrients will aid the process, while a low calorie count loaded with fats and sugars will slow it—but the weight will go.

The truth is, many people who battle the bulge kid themselves about how much they are eating in a day. They nibble while they prepare a meal, graze while the water is heating for tea, and take "just a few" of the candies in the candy dish at work—the five to ten times that they walk by it in a day. The portions that they eat at meals are consistently above the standard guide for healthful eating. And they have somehow bought the argument that if the cookie is broken, the calories have fallen out. They may also neglect to count the average one hundred calories for every tablespoon of oil or dressing on a salad, the fifty to one hundred calories for every helping of butter on toast or potato, and the added calories in that guilt-free cup of coffee every time that they pour in the half-and-half and stir in the sugar.

If you truly want to get your weight under control, be honest with yourself about how much you eat. Long-term habits of unconscious eating can be difficult to break. The best solution is a short-term commitment to tracking every bite. Carry a notepad and pen with you for one week. Every time you put *anything* in your mouth, write it down. That means all the extras, too—not just the main attractions. Sauces, cheese toppings, condiments, butter, oil, salad dressings, jams, honey, sugar, syrup, and nuts—all of these embellishments and others count, and how much of them you add counts. Notice what comes with restaurant meals and what the portion sizes are. They all count.

If you really want to reckon with the consequences of your eating habits, take the time not only to make an accurate record of what you are eating, but also to look up calorie and fat content so that you see what your food choices mean in relation to weight loss. Perhaps the exercise of recording and counting food intake won't ultimately change your habits, but at least you'll be living in the real world. You'll know that it is no mystery why you don't lose the weight that you want.

13.

Forgive Yourself

We are all really much more than the sum of our parts. The mind, body, emotions, and spirit all work as part of a system, interacting in ways that the most accomplished of experts have yet to entirely discover. So perhaps it is not surprising that our attitudes about ourselves have a profound effect on what we do and how we do it.

This is certainly evident in the realm of weight loss. Such statements as "I don't have time to exercise," or "I'm addicted to chocolate," all represent attitudes that easily translate into self-defeating behavior. We have an idea of ourselves in our heads and actually make it happen. On an insightful day, we call it self-fulfilling prophecy.

We defeat ourselves in a more subtle way when we make a plan for weight loss, put ourselves to the task, see results, and then "fall off the wagon" for some reason. Maybe it's a family visit for the holidays, a lavish event, or a vacation. Maybe it's just a lack of will on a gloomy afternoon. The reason is immaterial. What counts is what we do with the potential disappointment in ourselves after we indulge. For some, such a lapse leads to self-hatred, discouragement, or fatalism. They let one lapse lead to another, asking, "What's the use in trying?" Or they put such emphasis on the "failure" that they cease to focus on the path and results of success.

We all have days when our best-laid plans go awry. We are, after all, human, subject to changes and influences, from both within and without, that we cannot predict. On the plus side of the equation is our ability to effect change, and no more powerful engine of change exists than our attitude. If we're down on ourselves and lose confidence in our power to make a difference in our lives, we can actually cause the behavior that will short-circuit our hopes and goals. If, on the other hand, we recognize the certainty of lapses in the most disciplined routines, and have the generosity and wisdom to forgive ourselves when they occur, we stand in a far stronger position to get right back to doing what serves our best interests. We can learn from the mistakes and adjust for more success.

The moral of the story is this: You really are only human. You will make mistakes and do what you don't want to do sometimes. But your ability to change for the better is only enhanced by experiences—good and bad. You can learn, you can grow, and you can become more and more of what you want to be. Forgive yourself the lapses of behavior. Live and learn, get over it, and get on with what you want to do.

14.

Distinguish Food from Love

In our earliest days of existence, we experience two needs that must be met for our survival. One is the need for nourishment, the other for loving physical contact. For many of us, both needs are amply met in those early days almost exclusively by our mothers or mother-surrogates. In fact, many of us come to closely associate mother love, and later self-love, with the business of being fed. Since adequate nourishment continues to serve our survival and well-being, we shouldn't be surprised by that association.

If, however, we struggle with overeating or eating when we are not hungry, we may need to reckon with the love-food connection in a direct, conscious way. Eating *in order to feel loved* often grows out of depression and low self-esteem. But many of the foods that attract people seeking a quick "pick-me-up" are high in sugar and fat, and they actually work against the need to feel better in the long run. They detract from a well-balanced approach to diet, and often lead to weight gain, poor self-image, and mood swings.

You can certainly love yourself through the way that you care for yourself, but not by raiding the cookie jar, eating more than you need, or answering every negative mood with an oral fix. Rather, consider how much of your eating is emotionally driven. If, with reflection, you find that you are eating to recreate mother love in your life, apply some common sense to the formula. Worthy mother love keeps your best interests always at heart. Part of caring well for yourself is eating in a way that keeps you at a healthy weight with a maximum of vitality. Plenty of guides exist to spell out in detail what such a diet consists of.

When you need a lift or a little love, try turning to other sources of self-care. Take a long walk, indulge in an hour of your favorite reading, make a date with someone whose company you enjoy, or sign up for a course of study that interests you and enhances your life. Take action that takes the whole of your needs into account. Over time, with some awareness and imagination, you will find that you have moved on from the infant-style equation of food with love.

15.

Watch Food-Centered Socializing

Food has always taken center stage in many social situations. Gathering with friends or family is often about sharing meals, cooking together, and enjoying the indulgences inherent in many mealtime rituals. Making food the *raison d'être* of your socializing is easy to do, but hard to keep under control.

All sorts of opportunities exist to focus on food for fun. Great restaurants have never appeared with more frequency, nor have they had more attention than now. With a diversity of cultures in modern society, trying food from every background and ethnicity has come to hold a prime position in the list of things to do with friends. We have to eat, after all, and doing it in style with friends is not a bad option. It can become a problem, however, when it starts taking over the social calendar. It is an easy road to overindulging in rich, fattening food and alcohol. Even the most disciplined eater can feel that it's rude or lacking in spirit to opt out of the indulgences offered at a friendly gathering. For anyone who struggles with self-control, it can spell disaster.

Measure how much socializing you do that includes or centers around eating. You don't have to forsake such socializing, but in the interest of weight loss or control, you may do yourself a big favor by limiting it. Like virtually everything in life, moderation is a good idea. In fact, moderation can heighten your enjoyment of these events. They will become special events to revel in. Remember that you always have choices, and they are yours alone to make.

16.

Fashion Models Make
Poor Role Models

The myth of thinness as either the norm or the epitome of beauty has come and gone through the ages, and perhaps most especially through the twentieth and into the twenty-first century. Today, it makes its most ubiquitous appearance in advertising campaigns for hundreds of product lines, from high fashion to household appliances to automobiles. Whatever the product, advertisers have learned that there is no more powerful message than "If you buy this, you'll look like this."

Like it or not, those advertising experts are paid to know how to sell, however deceptively, and they know their business. As you watch commercial television, read magazines, or drive along well-traveled roads, you are bombarded by a steady stream of effective campaigns carrying messages that thin equals beautiful, successful, and happy.

Read the stories from behind the scenes and you'll find out differently. Fashion models are among those at highest risk for eating disorders. Behind those so-called perfect bodies are a myriad of well-documented issues of substance abuse and self-esteem issues. Many models in fashion and advertising have to focus their entire attention on the appearance of things, rather than the substance. Looks are doomed to fail us, over time. Character, good relationships, good health, and meaningful involvement in work and play can last a lifetime.

The problem is that we sometimes take in the message without even realizing it. The image of the young, thin, and glamorous lodges deep in our psyches without conscious effort or evaluation. We go to a store to buy new garments with such visions in our heads and suffer agonies over what appears in the dressing room mirror. We put ourselves together for a workday or an evening out and leave home dispirited because we haven't measured up to an ideal that we've imbibed when we weren't aware of it.

Weight control has real and important ramifications for good health and quality of life, but reaching and maintaining a healthy weight for your particular age and body bears no relation at all to what you see in the ads. You probably cannot avoid the unrealistic weight messages. In modern society, they are all around you. You can, however, become conscious of their effectiveness and build a new self-awareness in response to them. Thinness can't hold a candle to a healthy mind and body.

17.

Pay Attention to Quantity

Let's face it: What you eat matters when it comes to weight control. An entire industry has been built around this fact. What is most interesting, however, in the present age of diet soda, no-fat goodies, and numerous weight-loss programs and publications is the concurrent, dramatic rise in obesity. How can we explain this?

Certainly, part of the problem stems from people who make a habit of eating high-fat and high-sugar food, fast food, and an overload of nutrition-poor packaged food, despite all of the information on the negative effects of such a diet. There is also the matter of quantity. Anyone who eats out with any regularity has observed that the average restaurant plateful could easily be divided into two or three adequate meals for a moderate eater. People in the United States, especially, tend toward a diet that provides a much higher proportion of meat protein than anywhere else in the world—an amount that is fattening, not necessary for good health, and can actually lead to disease. The standard advice on portion size is to eat a piece of meat, fish, or poultry no larger than a fist, and at least several meals a week that replace meat foods with vegetable protein combinations.

It has also become apparent that people eat low- or no-fat food in far larger portions than necessary because they believe the lack of fat means quantity no longer matters. Wrong. This is true, as well, with the "diet" desserts and snacks. True, they often contain less fat or sugar, but they still have calories. Just because the box touts the food as "diet" does not mean that you can down the whole contents without fear of gaining weight.

Even if you are eating a well-balanced combination of good foods, you only need so much. Your doctor or health professional can give you an educated idea of how many calories will make a reasonable total per day for your size, gender, age, and activity level. Combine that with the aforementioned well-rounded diet, and you will soon take yourself off of the list of the newly overweight. No tricks. No frills. Just common sense. Don't eat more than you need to eat.

18.

Know the Truth About Nutrition

There's really no excuse in the modern world for ignorance about good eating habits. If anything has received adequate attention from health experts for all age groups, it's nutrition. In fact, a standard guide to human nutritional needs has been published by the U.S. government and reproduced on the side or back panels of many kinds of food packaging. We don't lack for information about nutrition, but it won't help us unless we look for it, seek to understand it, and put it to good use in our own daily eating habits.

Remember that your body needs a complicated balance of nutrients to function efficiently and healthfully. One of the obvious problems with eating food that is poor in nutrients is that it does not meet those needs. Your health and well-being suffer, and the resulting imbalance may contribute to a weight problem, as well as numerous other health-related difficulties. A less obvious side effect of eating poorly is that because you are not getting the nutrients that you need, your body continues to demand food. You feel a desire to eat despite the fact that you've consumed as many or more calories than you require. You continue to eat, but it does not satisfy the real needs that your apparent hunger represents. So you eat more. And so on. You can readily imagine where this cycle leads.

This happens, as well, with fad diets that focus on a limited variety of foods. Aside from the boredom factor that almost invariably sets in, your body knows what it is missing. When you're eating out of balance for some quick-loss weight plan, you eventually reach the point at which physical and psychological deprivation set in and lead to overeating.

Don't allow a lack of knowledge about nutrition to subvert your hopes for a healthy, fit body. Read up on the subject. Get to know what the current, medically sound wisdom on different food is. If you have particular food challenges—allergies, intolerances, or disease-related diet requirements—make them a focus of concentrated study until you know the facts well enough that they become second nature to you. Once you have the information, put it to the test. Make a commitment to practicing an eating style that reflects what you have learned, even if only for a month. You can be sure that if you replace a nutrition-poor diet with one that follows informed guidelines, you will experience positive returns in vitality, weight control, and self-esteem.

19.

Account for Different
Eaters at Home

One of the challenges of living with other people is accommodating different tastes and habits. This is as true in the area of eating as in any other, whether it has to do with tidiness, choice of television programs, or how you squeeze the toothpaste tube. Whether you're dealing with a family or a housemate situation, eating differences can land you with challenges and temptations that you'd rather not have.

Challenges and temptations appear whenever you're trying to institute or maintain any good habit. When they do, it's easy to turn them into handy excuses for letting your good resolve slip. The only antidote is personal honesty. The fact that you face temptation does not mean that you have to give in. When you give in, you have made a choice, pure and simple. Face it, reckon with it, and keep in mind that your next choice does not have to be the same. Putting to the test what will serve your long-range goals does not have to become the first step to abandoning those goals. Rather, it gives you an opportunity to build character and strength of purpose and to exercise good habits that will serve you for a lifetime.

Be realistic, as well as honest. If you have children in the house or your partner or housemate happens to love or need food that is off your preferred list, you may have to find ways to deal with the presence of such food. You don't always have the option of insisting that everyone should eat the way that you want to eat. Strategize. Whenever possible, make the food that serves your goals the easiest to reach and see. Separate the items that don't belong in your diet, and find a storage place for them that is off your beaten path. If you're cooking for or eating with people who eat in ways that don't work for you, be prepared to have some separate dishes for yourself. It's easy today to cook a quantity of good food ahead and store it in individual servings that can be defrosted or reheated in short order.

You do not need to be victim of other people's preferences or needs. Know yourself. Know what you're aiming for. Think ahead, and take the steps that will let you be both prepared and proactive in the face of challenges and temptations. You will be well rewarded.

20.

Learn How to Stop Eating

It could be argued that the major cause of otherwise healthy individuals being overweight is eating beyond the point of satiation. We eat between meals, even when we aren't hungry. We take seconds when we've had enough. We clean our plates, even though our dietary needs have been satisfied. There are probably many reasons why we keep eating when we ought to stop. The trick is to identify the reasons and take steps to change the habits that have resulted.

For example, many of us were raised in families in which we were told that leaving food was wasteful, that it would insult the cook, or that we wouldn't grow strong without every last crumb. It's amazing how that early training settles into our psyche for a lifetime.

In addition, we may perpetuate habits that developed at an earlier or different time in our lives. As growing children, we often needed between-meal energy boosters. Our calorie needs were high and our activity was constant. Maybe we formed the habit of grabbing something midmorning or midafternoon, or we routinely helped ourselves to dessert. We continue that style of eating, not because our needs have remained the same, but because the habits have pleasant associations with youth or family.

Of course, many of us simply eat too fast. We're always in a hurry and gobble what's put in front of us. As a result, our systems do not have time to register that we've consumed what we need, and we keep eating.

Whatever the reason that you eat after you should stop, identify it and work to learn better strategies. If you have a compulsion to eat everything on your plate, put less on your plate in the first place. Forget seconds. If someone else serves you, either tell the person to go light on the portions, or learn to understand that eating more than you need is a great deal more wasteful (in every sense of the word) than leaving some food behind.

If you eat too fast, become conscious of chewing your food thoroughly. Develop the habit of replacing utensils on the plate between bites. A half-hour before mealtime, drink a large glass of water so that you don't approach a meal with a ravenous appetite or an empty feeling in your stomach.

These are simple strategies. They require a little self-knowledge and a clear view of what you want in the long run. It's not a big deal to learn how to stop eating, but it is a learning process.

21.

Reconsider Your Heroes

Whom do you admire most? What draws you to such an individual? What characteristics or attitudes make him or her stand out? What specifically would you emulate?

Such questions have much to reveal about self-esteem. Most of us carry at least a short list of heroes, present or past, who embody some qualities that we find estimable. Yet we rarely focus on these people and their qualities when we are evaluating ourselves. We are immersed in a world that gives inordinate attention to the superficial. It's no wonder that we place so much stock in achieving the perfect weight when we're inundated with the message that our physical appearance matters more than anything else.

The place that weight loss and control play in your life reflects, to some extent, what you value about yourself. But unless your list of heroes is filled with people whose business first and foremost is to look good, your weight concerns may not reflect what you truly esteem in others. Without much thought, you may be buying into more superficial values instead of keeping issues of physical beauty in their place while you pursue more valuable interests.

Review your heroes. Pay attention to what they do that warrants your admiration. Then reconsider what you choose to occupy your time and thoughts. Reaching and maintaining a reasonable weight has its place, certainly, for the sake of good health and quality of life, but it hardly warrants center stage when compared to character, relationships, and meaningful activity.

22.

Make Allowances for
Special Occasions

Consistent attention to how you eat and exercise makes an enormous difference in effectively losing and maintaining weight. It takes a regimen of good habits to stay off the weight roller coaster. But we all know that even with the best habits and strongest resolve, we sometimes find ourselves in situations in which staying with our regimen seems disappointing. A fabulous meal, a high-spirited celebration, or a one-time event can lose its luster if you feel that you can only experience it with a relentlessly applied weight program firmly in place.

No weight battle was ever lost because of the rare special occasion. If you honestly stick with a reasonable plan of diet and exercise most of the time, you won't undo the good results with a single event's enjoyment. But remember that this truth depends on two elements. First, you really do make a healthful regimen the rule, day after day, week after week. It needs to be your way of life, not an on-again, off-again band-aid to self-defeating habits. Second, the special occasion has to be rare. If you're attending special events several times a week, you need to get honest with yourself. That's not the exception; it's part of the rule.

Once you learn to balance a healthful lifestyle with the occasional special time, you may also find ways to plan ahead and make allowances for such a time. Adding extra exercise can offer you leeway when it's time to relax your regimen. Giving yourself a couple of "light" days on the eating side of the equation can sometimes free your conscious and your constitution for the rich food that you don't ordinarily include in your eating. You'll enjoy yourself more and avoid the disappointing aftermath of overindulging.

Remember that life is more than regimens, but regimens can add quality to life. You don't have to forsake self-control in order to have a good time. Neither does fun have to undo the satisfying results of steady good-health habits. Pace yourself so that the special occasions remain special. Understand what you can do to enjoy them responsibly and without guilt. Life is too short to let happy occasions pass us by or undermine our goals.

23.

Postpone Indulgences

How many times have you spoken the words, "Tomorrow. The diet definitely begins tomorrow," to yourself? After which you help yourself to one more serving of that Super Fudge Nutty Crunch ice cream that won't be denied. Best-laid diet plans safely put aside, you declare yourself free to indulge and subvert your hopes to get weight and eating under control for another day. Unfortunately, "tomorrow" easily becomes a habit. One tomorrow follows another, and before you know it, a month of tomorrows has passed and you're no closer to strengthening your resolve. The only progress that you've made is in the level of frustration that you feel with yourself.

Most of us procrastinate at one time or another. When some unwanted challenge arises, we look for any excuse to help us postpone the necessary. If this has been your *modus operandi* for most of your life, you're not likely to oust the attitude immediately, or even once and for all. The procrastination mindset is notoriously hard to lose—but you may be able to learn how to refocus it.

For just one day, try turning the tables on your urge to put off. Instead of postponing control of what and how much you eat, try telling the treat to wait—just for today. Tell yourself, "just for today," day by day for a week or two, and you'll have made a good start on reaching your goal. Your daily success will gain momentum and help motivate you for each day going forward. You'll be on the way to gaining an excellent tool for managing procrastination in other areas of your life.

24.

Find the Art in Food

Food is a gift for our sustenance and physical satisfaction, certainly—but it's also a gift for our senses. Just consider the amazing variety that exists in each of the food groups. Work your way, for example, through the produce department of any food store and take in the array of shapes, sizes, colors, and consistencies of just one category of food. Something as plain as root vegetables offers up a fascinating variety: potatoes that are white, purple, red, or brown, sweet or savory; deep purple beets, orange carrots, white and lavender turnips, beige parsnips, and golden rutabagas; crisp and pungent celery roots and fennel. Move on to vegetables that grow on vines, bushes, or stalks; in heads or as bulbs. Meander through the bins of fruit large as melons or tiny as wild blueberries. While you're at it, take in the intensity of the fresh herbs and dried spices.

It's a paradise of plenty for sight, touch, taste, and smell, and we take it for granted, more often than not. What a shame to lose the pleasure of the beauty and variety that we've been given.

You can learn to take your time with food if you can teach yourself to pay attention to its intrinsic beauty. When you begin to take an interest in the possibilities that the raw materials offer, you can begin to slow down the rest of the food business in your life. Take more time to select what you eat, and then enjoy making meals with it that live up to the beauty and flavor of the medium. You will eventually become someone who wouldn't dream of stuffing your mouth on the run, because you savor the pleasure of sitting down to the food that you've chosen and prepared with real appreciation. Life is short. Food is necessary. Why not make an art of it?

25.

Deal with Secret Eating

O kay, be honest. Do you sneak into the kitchen when no one else is around to take a giant spoonful of ice cream, to shave off another slice of pie, or to slather some peanut butter on a cracker? You don't have to tell anyone else, but you need to admit it to yourself if you're hiding what and when you eat. If you're eating in secret, it's almost certainly because you're eating quantities or kinds of food that you know are not in your best interest. Every time that you tiptoe to the pantry and gobble the goodies, you're choosing to cheat yourself of all that you might be and do in regard to diet and weight control. The closet-eating habit can be a difficult one to break. Unless or until you admit what you're doing, at least to yourself, it will be impossible to stop.

Learning to overcome secret eating isn't an end in itself. It's simply one of a number of steps that you can take to accept responsibility for your own health and well-being. There are many circumstances and events in life over which we have no control. What and how much you choose to eat are absolutely in your control.

If this is a problem for you, begin by ruthlessly writing down every secret bite that you take. You may be fooling yourself that it really isn't *that* much extra food. When you actually keep track, however, you'll teach yourself to be more aware of what you're doing and what the consequences of it are.

Once you get honest with how much you're eating and when, consider enlisting a friend who can be your buddy in overcoming the habit. Sometimes, simply having someone to talk to can give you the motivation to do what will give you long-term satisfaction. If the person that you choose is a close friend, you may even agree to call each other when the urge to eat in secret comes over you. Instead of reaching into the cookie jar, reach for the phone and say, "Help!" A good friend can be your willpower when your own determination flags.

Secret eating doesn't have to be a big deal. Once you admit it, it ceases to be a secret. Once you start making conscious, self-loving choices instead of giving into self-defeating impulses, you'll discover the joy of taking charge of your own life and welfare.

26.

Lose the Movie Star Ideal

So what? You're not the physical equal of the latest celebrity heartthrob? You can't match the angles and curves of the breathtaking leading lady? You don't have the rippling abs and rugged jawline of the dashing hero? Join the crowd.

It's time to get real. Granted, we live in an age of glamour and hype, designed to sell tickets, magazines, and clothes. But while we're consuming entertainment and products, we don't have to buy into the myth that what we see in the media is realistic or ideal for most of us. That road leads to misery for too many people today. We deprive ourselves, feel guilty every time that we break a diet, develop eating disorders, and hate ourselves every time that we stand before dressing-room mirrors.

Perhaps you think that if only you looked like a celebrity, you could make a greater success of your everyday life. Or maybe you think that it would grant you great pleasure and satisfaction to turn heads wherever you go. Think again.

Take a long, honest look at what you know of the lives of the extraordinary beauties of our age. Notice how frequently their relationships come apart at the seams. Pay attention to their reactions to the relentless invasions of their privacy. Imagine how they must feel when one after another unwanted advance is inflicted on them. Consider how difficult it is for them when time takes its toll on their chief asset, physical beauty.

Real life is not a movie. Real people come in all shapes and sizes. Your ultimate happiness does not depend on the exterior that you were born with. It depends on who and what you are, what you value, and what you do about it. Go ahead and buy that ticket. Sit back and enjoy the fantasy for an hour or two. But don't rob yourself of the enjoyment that you can derive from your own unique set of qualities. You are who you are. Make the most of it.

27.

Replace Processed
Food with Whole

Statistics seem to support the observation that as a nation, we are gaining weight. Many theories have been advanced as to what might be causing this phenomenon, but experts seem to agree that at least one of the culprits is processed, packaged food products. As we have become more affluent, urban, and industrialized, we have moved farther away from the sources of our food and from food in its natural state.

First, we eat food additives without knowing that we're doing so. Many processed foods include extra salt and sugar to enhance flavor. Because fat also enhances the taste of food, it finds its way into our typical food products. The simplest, most wholesome of raw ingredients come through the processing with a remarkably altered sugar and fat content, and that means that we are taking in many more calories than we can reasonably burn in a day.

Second, we eat food that has often been milled or processed to the point that its natural balance of nutrients and structural characteristics has been lost. The fiber that helps to make us feel full after eating and aids in the digestive process is substantially reduced. The natural vitamins and minerals, often destroyed in the processing, are replaced by synthesized versions of the same, and in quantities quite unlike what occur in the food naturally. It's quite possible that we feel like we want to go on eating when we've ingested more than enough calories, in part because we haven't taken in an equal quantity of the nutrients that we need for good health.

Third, we eat food in prepackaged quantities, whether in take-home entrees or in restaurants, that far exceed what we need or can use. The standard wisdom among health experts on a suitable serving of meat or fish, for example, is approximately four ounces. Yet it's the rare restaurant that doesn't offer a massive portion of meat or chicken. Add to that the largest possible potato with the equivalent of three average pats of butter, a bowl piled with pasta, a salad loaded with dressing, a basket of bread, and you've got yourself a weight problem waiting to happen.

There's nothing wrong with a good, prepared meal, but if that's what you eat most of the time, your weight-control efforts will be Herculean. Try making whole foods, simply prepared, as your meals of choice. Let the processed foods be the exception. You'll notice a difference in how you feel and how you look. And you may discover that the food in its closer-to-natural state doesn't need all the additives and processing to make it tasty and satisfying.

28.

Take the "Diet" Out of Your Diet

There are many places in the world today where people would scratch their heads at our western notions of "going on a diet." Food supplies are scarce, and having enough to eat to survive is sometimes in question. For most of us in modern societies, survival is not an issue. Instead, we refer to "diet" when we intend to restrict or otherwise manage our intake or choice of food in order to lose weight.

The problem with this choice of language, and its connotation, is that we build a mentality around the idea of "diet" that becomes negative. We think of ourselves, on a diet, as being deprived. Because we think in terms of foods that we cannot eat on a diet, we come to long for those foods. They seem to call us from the cupboard, refrigerator, or deli counter.

In fact, the old-fashioned meaning of "diet" refers to habitual eating patterns. Farmers ate a diet of homegrown produce and meat. Island peoples had a diet derived from the sea. Arctic populations ingested a diet high in animal fat.

Now consider the potential difference in mindset if you were to shift your sense of diet from the former, restrictive connotation to the latter idea meaning eating habits. In the interest of weight control and general good health, you might decide to focus on a diet higher in fiber, lower in animal fats, and loaded with fresh, whole foods—especially vegetables and fruits. Unlike the negative thrust of being "on a diet," this carries a positive message of caring for yourself and enjoying good fresh foods. Instead of feeling deprived, you'll feel cared for and privileged.

This is not a trick. It's the truth of what such eating habits are and produce in you. The difference isn't just in the way you say it, or how you construe it, although both are meaningful in terms of your attitude. The difference is in what you're doing for yourself when you eat healthfully.

29.

Make Accommodations for Kids

It's all very well to decide that you are going to change your eating habits in the interest of weight control and related health issues. It's another thing altogether to deal with it realistically when you've got growing kids at home. Healthy, active kids burn calories like mad, and in this age of very effective advertising, they tend to gravitate toward the high-sugar, high-fat junk foods available. If you give them what they want, you're likely to have food in the house that you'd rather not have.

A couple of thoughts: First of all, healthful, low-fat, and low-sugar snack food does exist. You don't have to settle for the refined sweets or fatty stuff that derail your good intentions and are probably responsible for an unprecedented level of obesity in today's children. Fresh fruit is always a winner. So, too, are whole-wheat tortillas topped with a reduced-fat cheese and broiled, then cut into homemade tortilla "chips" and offered with some salsa. A moderate amount of natural peanut butter on apple slices or celery sticks, trail mixes made with nuts and dried fruit, yogurt with sliced bananas, or whole wheat toast and fruit-only preserves can serve as a satisfying and sustaining afternoon mini-meal that doesn't rely on refined carbohydrates or fats, or an excess of salt for flavor.

Second, kids learn to enjoy wholesome snack foods and well-rounded meals when that is what's offered. Generally speaking, if they are allowed a regular diet of junk foods, they'll develop a preference for those foods. If their choices are limited to the healthy ones, they'll find their preferences among the good stuff.

Third, your children's welfare is closely linked to yours. If you're happy and healthy, they'll benefit. If you feed them the way that you know you should feed yourself, they'll learn habits that will become life skills when they're older.

30.

Plan for Maintenance

A lot of us know how to lose weight when we need to. We *should* know how. We've done it dozens of times. We're pros at the weight-loss game. But the reason that we've had to repeat the process so many times (with increasing difficulty as time goes by, it should be said) is because while we know how to lose, we're short on understanding when it comes to maintaining an optimum weight.

The challenge goes back to our conception of "diet." We often think of weight-reduction plans rather than of new habits of eating. As long as you're of a mind to put yourself on a "weight-loss" program—which is to say, a diet that cannot be sustained because it lacks balance or sufficient calories to satisfy your physical requirements—you'll run into trouble when you reach your target size and shape. Having achieved the goal, you'll fall back into what you consider to be "normal" eating. The problem is that the "normal" way of eating is what landed you in the situation of needing to lose weight in the first place.

You'll put yourself a giant step ahead of the game if you recognize ahead of time that on the slim side of the weight-loss challenge, you still have to think about how you eat. The very same types of food that helped you lose will help you maintain your new weight. You'll probably be able to eat a moderately increased volume of food, or you'll be able to add an occasional treat. But in essence, how and what you eat for the sake of trimming down is exactly what's needed to remain trim.

Do your homework before you launch a weight-control plan in your life. Make sure that what you're planning is healthy enough that you can make it a permanent way of life without threat to your physical well-being. Pay attention to satisfying your need for flavor and variety. You do yourself an enormous disservice when you use an eating plan that leaves you bored, hungry, or craving favorite snacks. The more you concentrate on finding whole foods that you like and learning how to cook these foods to maximize their flavor and health benefits, the more likely you are to establish a lifelong set of good eating habits that will ensure that your weight-loss days are at an end.

31.

Keep the Whole Person in View

Clichés are usually rooted in truth. "You are what you eat" certainly is. What we eat becomes the building material for our physical selves, and has a profound effect on our health, moods, appearance, and energy.

Yet when we are intent on losing weight, what we eat may take on disproportionate importance. So much emphasis is placed on food in our culture, and on "diet" foods and programs in the media, that we forget that what we are and what we do about weight control is linked to much more than food intake. We often forget that losing weight is not the answer to all of our problems, nor is it the ultimate source of peace and joy.

We think of exercise in the same way. Research has shown that exercise—movement of all sorts—offers great benefits for overall wellness, and specifically for weight management. As the positive benefits of a regular, moderate level of activity that raises heart rate and tones muscles become clear, more attention is being given to exercise programs. This is good and will certainly help us with weight issues, but it still doesn't account for how complex we humans really are.

The truth is that we are more than just physical beings, and life is more than weight control. We have intellectual needs for mental challenge and stimulation, and spiritual needs for love, friendship, and nurturing. We want and need connections to other people, to nature, and to God or the transcendent. The frustrations that we experience related to maintaining a physical appearance that pleases us are often symptomatic of deeper needs than those related to physical appearance. When we concentrate our efforts on the physical and neglect the intellectual, emotional, spiritual, or psychological, we do ourselves a disservice.

When you're fretting over whether or how or when you'll lose extra weight, stop and consider what else in your life may need your loving attention. Don't forget that you are a wonderfully complicated organism with personality, temperament, pains, pleasures, fears, and hopes. It is up to you to take care of your physical well-being. Keep the whole of you in mind.

32.

Identify Your Eating Triggers

Most of us who have struggled with extra weight have to admit on an honest day, that the extra weight comes from eating extra food—that is, food beyond what we need to meet our nutritional and energy needs. Some of us realize after a few unsuccessful stabs at self-control that we often eat extra food for reasons other than physical hunger or thirst. A few of us know what those reasons are.

Understanding is the first step toward making the conscious choices about your eating habits that will give you the results you want. Keeping track of time, place, mood, food choice, and even your emotions when you indulge in overeating can be remarkably revealing. You may discover that you have a hunger spurt at the same between-meal time every day that relates to what you ate at the previous meal. You may then decide to change that meal's intake, or to build in a planned snack that keeps the eating under control and within the framework of your goals.

On the other hand, you may find that when you feel like eating extra, you're responding to a mood more than a physical hunger.

Maybe you're bored, frustrated, or a little blue. Maybe you feel restless and need to move around, so you head in the direction of the kitchen out of habit. If this is the case, you can teach yourself new responses. Whether it's getting out of the house for a walk, calling a friend for a talk, taking a soothing bath, or simply switching gears to do something else, you can plan ahead and try any number of substitutes until you find some that work for you.

Of course, we all have long-term associations of eating with certain activities, times, or events. Some people grow up in a household in which the standard fare in the evening is watching the television with snack food close at hand. Others have their best family times around a game board with snack bowls abounding. When you eat more than you want or need, you may be reliving pleasurable moments from your past. Once you know this, you should be able to choose differently.

The point is that knowing what triggers your eating gives you a vital tool for change. Pay attention and take responsibility for the choices that you're making. Don't kid yourself into thinking that you can't help yourself when the urge to eat hits. You can change your behavior. The first step is recognizing it, and the next is understanding it.

33.

Replace "Good/Bad" Language

There's something paradoxical about the "good/bad" language that we often associate with eating, especially when we're trying to control our weight. It's "good" when we say "no" to some tempting treat. It's "bad" when we eat something that isn't part of the plan. Oddly enough, when we're "good," it's often grudgingly accomplished. When we're "bad," we get some pleasure out of jumping off course. In other words, it's bad to be "good," and it's good to be "bad."

Rather than think in terms of good and bad behavior in relation to food, think in terms of good health and vitality. Imagine your organs operating at peak efficiency, your muscles growing strong and lean, and your energy at optimal level. You may just find that some fresh fruit suits your mood better than a doughnut.

It's hard to overestimate the value and influence of attitude. When we throw the food choices that we make into the arena of "good" and "bad," we take on a self-hating attitude that can only rob us of satisfaction in the present and of hope in the future.

34.

Play with Your Food

Remember when you were a kid? Did you ever make an igloo out of your mashed potatoes? Or pour the pancake batter in the shape of Mickey Mouse's head? There was a level of play and imagination in that activity that is lost later in life. Perhaps you were told once too often, "Stop playing with your food!" You got it into your head that food and eating are serious, no-nonsense business, and you lost interest in being creative.

Well, resurrect that playfulness that fed your imagination in childhood. If your eating patterns have sagged into a sameness that keeps the pounds on and your mood depressed, you can choose to change—and change can begin with a sense of adventure.

There's more than enough printed material available, and a number of cable television shows, that show us new ways to prepare food that tastes great without a lot of extra fat and calories. Three of the major components of these cooking styles are freshness, flavor, and presentation.

Adults who grew up in the 1950s, 1960s, and 1970s were barraged with packaged and frozen foods. We learned the true versatility of casseroles, ready-breaded food for frying, and mixes for all sorts of baked goods. Today, the emphasis has largely shifted, despite the ongoing orgy of packaged and precooked foods, to a broad variety of fresh foods that are available year-round. That abundance of fresh ingredients allows a home cook to make delicious, simple meals that still retain the texture and flavors of whole food.

You can add to the fresh ingredients a growing variety of available fresh herbs, hot peppers, quality olive oils (more flavor, so you can use less), international spices, and gourmet mustards and vinegars. Flavor is a huge factor in the enjoyment of food, and with many of the products now on the market, flavor is a ready option for keeping your food interesting without adding calories.

What's most fun with food preparation is the multitude of ideas for how to serve food so that it looks as enticing as it tastes. This is where playing with food becomes sheer pleasure. Check out the beautifully photographed cookbooks from your local library. Open to the lifestyles section of the newspaper, and you're likely to find one gorgeous food presentation after another. It doesn't take much to add a little color or dash to your dinner plate, but it offers a new zest for healthful, conscious eating.

You don't have to make every meal a masterpiece, but if you play with your food instead of accepting the tried and true, you can make the changes that will add pleasure without adding calories to your eating.

35.

Strategize for Food at Work

The workplace poses all kinds of challenges. For the weight conscious, these include power lunches, goodies that are set out for common consumption, snack bars, and vending machines. Add to that the sedentary nature of most office environments, and you've got yourself a challenge when it comes to eating and weight control.

Certainly the first step is taking responsibility for what you *do* with what is presented to you. Power lunches are sometimes important elements of the work dynamic, and there's no reason for you to take yourself out of that mix. Luckily, so many people are interested in taking control of their health and weight that virtually any restaurant offers alternatives to heavy, calorie- and fat-laden food. Look for "Heart Healthy" and "On the Light Side" on the menu, and you'll be moving in the direction of moderation. Remember, too, that you have no obligation to finish a meal that is oversized. Have it wrapped to go, or send it away with something left on your plate.

The tempting bowls of candy and plates of leftover birthday cake and pastry require a different strategy. If you feel deprived every time that you choose not to indulge, try the "everything in moderation" approach. Plan one goodie break at a prescribed time and take less than a full pastry, slice, or handful (you reach the last bite sooner or later—make it sooner). Don't make your treat a reward. Make the satisfaction of taking control the reward. You may eventually find that indulging doesn't attract you as much as limiting your indulgences.

As for the snack bars and vending machines, treat them with the disinterest that they deserve. Usually, all they offer is overpriced junk food, pure and simple. Instead of wasting your money and expanding your waistline, purchase an insulated snack bag to bring with you to work. Select some snacks at the supermarket or local produce stand that are good energy sources and satisfy the urge to chew—raw vegetable sticks, baby carrots, fresh fruit cut into bite-size pieces, dried fruit, bread sticks, or unbuttered popcorn, for example. Planning ahead allows you choices. Choices offer the opportunity to do and be what you want.

36.

Rise Above the Body Fads

If you believe that there is a perfect body type or ideal look, visit an art museum that offers art from a broad range of eras and cultures. The ideal has varied in amazing ways through the ages—and even in the last decade. Changes in what we associate with prosperity, the fashion industry's need for people to buy, and new findings about health are just a few of the factors that continue to keep us in a state of constant change. In truth, we're talking about fads—styles and perceptions that change with the passing of time.

You've already considered your body type. You understand that there are real limits to the sorts of adjustments that you can make to your general body traits. These have nothing to do with how much you weigh or how toned your muscles are. Yet like many others, you may forget body wisdom when the latest fad look explodes.

Be realistic. Look at yourself in the mirror. Remember what in your life has value that will last. Then think again about the latest fad and what trying to achieve it will add up to in your life. Is it worth it?

37.

Make Your Diet Well-Rounded

One of the many problems with fad diets is their tendency to focus on an eating plan that is neither balanced nor sustainable. This often leads to mood swings, irritability, boredom, feelings of deprivation, and a lack of good eating habits on the other side of weight loss. Many, many times, the next step is bingeing on all that you missed while on the diet. Before you know it, the weight is back on—and then some. Studies have shown that people who repeatedly lose and gain in this way have an increasingly difficult time losing.

Focusing your weight control efforts on a well-balanced eating plan takes off extra pounds slowly and naturally, and offers a sustainable way of eating and a greater sense of well-being in the meantime. The human body is a highly complicated system that requires chemical balance to operate efficiently. When you play around with the balance of what you ingest, you can wreak havoc on your metabolism. Your body has a great capacity to compensate and adjust, but there is often a price to pay over time in terms of psychological well-being and general health.

If you're fighting weight gain, you may not have a habit of well-balanced eating in the first place. Take advantage of the many available sources of information on what a well-balanced diet actually is. Health experts have provided ample advice, and there is substantial data to back up the wisdom of what they recommend.

Of course, all of the information in the world won't make you healthier or improve your eating habits. You have to take what you learn and put it into action. If your eating has been substantially out of whack, you may want to make a radical change that constitutes a fresh start. Make a plan, and put it into action. On the other hand, you may find it more successful to ease your way into new eating habits. Identify the particular habits that you need to change, and then choose just one a week that you will work on. This is a slow and steady process that may not yield dramatic results at first, but will produce real change over time.

38.

Know the Benefits of
Your Ideal Weight Range

Like body types, body weights vary among similar-sized people of different genders, ages, builds, and dispositions. The weight that is best for you probably falls within the range that doctors and researchers have determined for your combination of the above characteristics. If you don't already know where you should fall within that range, your doctor can certainly help you determine it. Knowing that piece of information is a good place to start whenever you're taking steps to lose or control your weight. It gives you a realistic goal and may provide extra motivation as you go.

Equally helpful is a clear sense of the value added to your life when you choose to reach and maintain a weight that is healthful for you. In our culture, the focus is almost always first and foremost on appearances. There's no denying that reaching your healthiest weight will contribute positively to your appearance—but that's just the obvious benefit. It isn't the most significant.

Maintaining a healthy weight means exactly that. Within your ideal range, you give your body all sorts of health advantages. You take weight-related strain off your vital organs, for starters. Information abounds on the negative effects of being overweight on the heart, for example. Many people don't realize that being overweight can also affect your circulatory system, your gall bladder, bladder, colon, and reproductive organs. Being overweight is also associated with increased risk of certain cancers.

When you keep the extra pounds at bay, you also do your joints a big favor. It's no surprise that with less weight to support, your joints take less stress, and you experience greater comfort and freedom of movement. In addition, being heavy has an adverse effect on such conditions as osteoarthritis.

Being overweight has also been implicated in respiratory ailments, sleep disorders, gout, and diabetes. Beyond the strictly physical, experts have identified numerous psychological difficulties that are related to carrying extra weight.

The upshot of all of the research is simply this: Every aspect of your physical, mental, and emotional well-being is affected by your weight. When you lose extra weight, you stand to gain greater health and happiness.

39.

Redefine "Wasted" Food

Many of us grew up mindful of the "starving children in faraway countries who didn't have any food on their plates." We're older now. We know perfectly well that licking the plate clean doesn't put food on the tables of those children. Certainly on the grand scale, the developed nations of the world could benefit from a greater conscience in relation to greed and misuse of the world's resources. Such a conscience will start with individuals like us who are the beneficiaries of plenty. It's appropriate that we take seriously wasting less, with an eye to making sure that there's plenty to go around.

However, once the food is on your plate, whether served up at home or in a restaurant, there are only two destinations for it: your stomach or the garbage pail. It is up to you to know what a reasonable portion of food for your size and activity level is. If you don't know, consider having a short conversation with your family doctor so that you do know. If you serve yourself, give yourself a single portion and stick with that. If someone else serves you, mentally or literally push aside anything more than the appropriate portions of each food. When the meal is over, let the extra go back to the kitchen.

It comes down to this: Any food served to you that is more than you need is *already* "wasted food." If you choose to eat it, it may very well also be "waisted." Which would you prefer?

40.

Identify Past Pitfalls

One of the great characteristics of the human mind is the capacity for memory and consequential thinking. As we live, we incorporate experience that provides us with essential information for a successful existence.

Make the most of this gift. Take the time to note the circumstances that send you off course in your weight-management plan. Do they include having certain types of food in the cupboard or refrigerator at home? What about skipping a meal? Or stopping at a certain bakery on the way home from work? Or choosing a certain restaurant for a meal out?

Whatever has turned out to be a pitfall in the past can be a learning tool for the present and future. Once you identify the times, places, and events that have been a challenge in the past, you can begin to strategize on ways to meet the challenge. You don't have to keep falling into the same holes. You can take different paths or build bridges. In other words, you can *learn* from your mistakes.

It is easier to move beyond problems in life when you learn to associate them with unwanted results. When you look back and see things you did that made you unhappy, reflect on the connection between your choices and the results of those choices. You're not a victim of circumstances. You can choose differently from what you chose in the past. You can take pitfalls and turn them into material for growth.

41.

Love Yourself in the
Way That You Eat

It's common to think that you're treating yourself to something special when you indulge in eating rich and decadent treats. For a few moments, your indulgence feels like a gift.

You're right that you deserve special treatment, and there's no reason why you shouldn't be the first one to extend loving gestures toward yourself. After all, the way that you care for yourself is the truest barometer of your self-esteem. It also often dictates the way that others will care for you. If you demonstrate that you love and respect yourself, others will often take their cue from you and treat you with similar love and respect.

Think again, though, about whether self-indulgence and self-love are the same thing. Would you consider it love if a friend tempted you with something that he or she knew you were trying to withstand? Far from an act of love, such treatment would almost rank as a betrayal. So, too, is laying aside your own good intentions for the sake of an impulsive surrender that doesn't take you closer to what you want to accomplish in and for yourself. Rather than respecting yourself enough to take the challenge seriously, you capitulate. For a critical moment, you shrug off your own best interests for the sake of a "treat," and almost invariably, the pleasure that results lasts a much shorter time than the regret that you feel soon after.

The same can be said for how you eat in general. You deserve the best-quality food, well prepared and eaten in healthful portions. Following a plan for eating that offers you optimal nutrition and health speaks of self-respect. Doing less than that—shoveling in whatever is easy or close at hand, for example, or eating on the run without attention to the food's beauty or value—shows a lack of self-respect.

It is a truer expression of self-love to look the consequences of how you eat square in the eye and say, "I deserve the best, not just for the moment, but for the long haul." When you do that, you love yourself in a meaningful way.

42.

Forget the Fad Foods

Fad foods are whatever edibles become the latest target in the world of marketing hype. A prime example in the last decade was the craze for pasta. Someone developed the notion that eating pasta, Mediterranean style, with plenty of vegetables, olive oil, and a good glass of wine, was unbeatable as a path to weight control and good health. This idea was based on statistics illustrating which populations worldwide showed the greatest resistance to heart disease and cancer and the least propensity to be overweight. There were, of course, some questionable assumptions about cause and effect in this particular fad. In addition, it disregarded the fact that the populations being touted as pasta beneficiaries actually grew the produce and made their pasta meals from fresh ingredients at home—and their activity levels were probably higher than those of most Americans. No one seemed to consider that these factors might be part of the reason that their diet had such a positive effect on their quality and length of life.

Unfortunately, some of the people looking for a magic bullet to cure the problem of being overweight latched on to the hype and missed some important fine print. Certainly, pasta with fresh vegetables and no animal fat has heart and health advantages over a diet heavy in red meat. But like any other type of diet, it is only effective if you eat it in moderation and balance it with other foods. Somewhere along the line, people got the impression that they could eat as much pasta as they wanted, as long as they stayed away from certain other foods. It's simply not true. Eat enough of anything—in short, eat more calories than you are burning—and you will gain weight.

This problem often arises with so-called "dietetic" foods, as well. A very lucrative business has grown up around the "lite" market. People read the "No fat!" banner or "Sugar-free" label, and think that they can binge at whatever rate they want. Despite the lack of sugar and fat, these fad foods still contain calories, and in many cases, contain precious little nutrients. The net result for consumers is a false impression that quickly backfires on them.

Forget the fad foods. Eating sensibly and moderately will give you many of the results that the fad-food sellers promise, and it will serve your long-term health and happiness far better.

43.

Use Food as Fuel

Food is fuel. It's what you run on, just as surely as a car runs on gasoline. Most of us know this, but we don't live it. We use food as comfort, luxury, reward, punishment, love, relief, and medicine. We preoccupy ourselves with it and build our days around its consumption. It takes on a disproportionate importance that makes it very difficult for us to put it in its place and keep it there when we're struggling with weight issues.

Never underestimate the power of your mind. You can retrain your way of thinking, just as you can change habits of hygiene, exercise, or sleep. In fact, in order to change *any* habit, whether breaking one or forming one, you must start with your inner thoughts. Begin by retraining how you perceive what you are doing and what you are going to do and that will direct your actions.

This is just as true with food habits as with any others. Your attitude has a profound effect on your behavior in relation to food. If you think of it as help in times of sadness or as reward in times of frustration, if you turn to it when you're bored or angry, you will eat when you are not hungry and pay the price for it in added pounds.

If, on the other hand, you plant in your mind the reality that food is primarily fuel, necessary for energy, growth, and repair, you can begin to understand the relevance of eating to keep yourself physically up and running. You can learn to eat when you're hungry and to not eat when you're not hungry. You can take into account the daily rhythms of your activities and the demands that they make on your system, and eat in a way that suits them. You can also learn to eat less when you do less, because you understand that you simply don't need as much fuel if you aren't covering as many miles.

Food as fuel doesn't require an undue amount of attention once you have a realistic sense of which foods, and how much, give you what you need. You can free your mind of food preoccupations, unlearn weight-challenging habits, and learn to deal with emotional issues in more productive and effective ways.

44.

A Healthy Relationship
with Your Scale

One of the dangers inherent in long-term battles with extra weight is an obsessive relationship with the scale. How many people with weight issues weigh themselves as soon as their feet hit the floor in the morning? In this way, they are likely to have the least amount of food and fluid in their bodies and apt to get the absolute lowest weight reading possible for the day. If the scale tips to the high side, a gloom cloud of self-hate and frustration settles over the day. If it registers on the low side, they perk up. In either case, the figures may be deceptive, and the very next day can show a difference of five pounds. No one gains or loses five pounds of real weight in a day, yet the scale can register such a change. So think twice before you invest too much emotional energy in the numbers.

The love-hate dynamic that develops around weighing in every day rarely has the desired effect of helping you adjust your eating habits to suit your needs. Instead, the anxiety and frustration that ensue from a "bad" weigh-in, or the false elation that comes from a "good" one, can load your eating decisions with enough emotional baggage to throw you into counterproductive behavior. You may be tempted to starve in the one case or overindulge in the other. Or you may simply carry around a weight-obsessed self-image that gets in the way of relationships and concentration. The extreme reaction for some can even be the beginning of something as serious and life-threatening as an eating disorder.

Many people have found that the best solution is to get rid of the bathroom scale, once and for all. They discover that they can develop a fairly accurate idea of what shape they're in without tying it to a specific number of pounds. By keeping it more general, they don't suffer over every fluky little shift in weight, and they are less likely to let weight issues assume overwhelming proportions. Some very successful weight-loss programs actually prescribe that people never weigh themselves at home, but rather wait for weekly or monthly "official" weigh-ins. In this way, they gain a far more accurate picture of the effect that their habits are having.

Move your scale out of sight and visit it less. It tells you something, but not everything, and its disadvantages easily "outweigh" its benefits.

45.

Beware the Gourmet Syndrome

Food magazines, cookbooks, and cooking shows are some of the hottest sellers on the market today, and restaurant eating has reached an unprecedented level. It's no wonder that we find ourselves thinking a lot about food—and not just any food, either. We're thinking about exotic food, special cuisines, reductions, sauces, stocks, and flourishes. We are living in the Age of Designer Food. This is not an unprecedented phenomenon. Many times throughout human history, civilizations have reached a level of prosperity that has made it possible to go to extremes in areas of pleasure.

Be that as it may, we're seeing a remarkable level of attention given to fancy eating. It's fun and delicious, but it can make weight control incredibly difficult. All of those wonderful oils, additives, and sauces tend to load on the fats and calories. It's not enough to have a lovely free-range chicken. You must wrap it in bacon, cozy it up to garlic mashed potatoes, and float it in a fat-laden sauce. Raspberries—a great food for the weight-conscious—show up in a sea of rich cream and doused with chocolate. These are feasts for the senses, but they take wholesome, low-calorie fresh foods and turn them into gourmet overindulgence.

You don't have to forego the trendy foods, but if you're interested in weight control, you'll need to seriously moderate your intake. It's fine to have a fling with some fine food once in a while, but balance it with a habit of simple eating most of the time. Your system can accommodate the occasional splurge, but it won't tolerate rich eating if it becomes the rule.

46.

Dress in Your Own Style

Be honest with yourself when you consider what you want to weigh. Are you aiming for a healthy, reasonable weight that falls within the range recommended by your doctor and other health experts? Or are you trying to achieve a weight that you believe will make it possible to don the latest fashion?

We could save ourselves a lot of misery if we came to terms with the fashion industry, once and for all. Designers make a living by coming up with new trends that tempt us all to run out and spend our money on new clothes long before our old ones have worn out. They are rarely concerned with the comfort of the buyer, and they apparently care not at all about whether the average body build will look good in what they invent. Their business is built on creating something different. That's the economy of fashion, and we would do well to it keep in mind when we're fretting over how we look in the latest styles.

Each of us has certain styles of clothing that do flatter our body types and suit our personal tastes. The styles may not be cutting edge.

In fact, the most flattering clothes tend to be what we term "classic" styles. They became classic precisely because they look good on a lot of different shapes and sizes. Conversely, we each have clothing styles that are decidedly not for us. Many of the fashions that could be termed "fads" fall into this category. They may be fun, whimsical, or extreme, but they flatter few figures, and they tend to last only a season or two.

If you enjoy experimenting with fashion, more power to you. But if your desire to do so leads you to fight against weight that is perfectly healthy for your body type and size, you may want to rethink the value of a season's passing fad. Is it worth the anguish that it causes? Finding fashions that flatter you when your weight is in the healthy range can ease tension. Choosing clothes that look good when you're carrying some extra pounds can safeguard your self-esteem while you make the changes needed to lose. Don't let the fashion world enslave you. You're the buyer. You're the boss. Choose to be happy.

47.

Understand Food and Mood

As has already been discussed, there is often a strong corollary between how we feel—our moods—and what we choose to eat. There is also scientific evidence that what we eat can affect our moods, for better or worse. A number of books and articles have been published in the last few years, putting forward various theories and eating plans designed to explain and capitalize on these effects.

It's all about common sense and the slow and steady effects of good health and nutrition. People who are in good health and a state of physical fitness experience a greater sense of well-being, generally speaking, than those who are not. With good health and healthy weight come vitality and an enhanced ability to perform well at work and play. Not surprisingly, that can be very good for your mood.

Eating a moderate, well-balanced diet of whole, fresh foods that have a minimum of fats and sugar in them is the only way to promote good health. Add to that regular, moderate exercise—which *has* been proven to have a beneficial effect on mood—and you have a simple, winning combination that has stood the test of time and experience.

It's important to understand how moods can tempt us to eat for comfort, because understanding it helps us to resist the counterproductive behavior. Eating to relieve emotional suffering is a false hope. The comfort is short-lived; the consequences of guilt, shame, and weight gain are not.

It's equally important to remember the positive effect that good nutrition and exercise will have on mood. Knowing the potential can provide the motivation that you need to develop eating and exercise habits that will pay lifelong dividends, not only for health, but also for happiness. It can't be repeated often enough. There are no quick fixes in life. Even miracle drugs take time, and they also take a toll in side effects. Improving the quality of your life in natural, common-sense ways may take longer, but it works, and it lasts.

48.

Feed Your Spirit

Man cannot live on bread alone. What we eat is one kind of nourishment, and we need it to survive, but it is not enough to sustain our spirit. One of the great shames of modern society's obsession with appearance is the extent to which it diverts us from tending to matters of character and spirituality. We get so hung up on how we look and what we weigh that we lose our sense of proportion. We get depressed over gaining a few pounds and neglect uplifting sources of encouragement and growth in great literature, philosophy, and religion. We're so intent on running off the latest weight gain that we forget to notice the beauty of nature all around us and the wonder of its rhythms and seasons.

Your spirit—your internal life—can be a great informer to the external. When you give serious attention to questions of meaning and purpose, you come to view questions of appearance and the superficial concerns of life in a different light. You begin to unburden yourself of standards imposed by others and gain the wisdom to think and choose what is important for yourself. You learn how to stand back and view the day-to-day worries from higher ground and put them into a larger, more encompassing context.

Don't let your time and attention be eaten up by immersion in the latest information on diet, exercise, fashion, or lifestyle. Take the days of your life seriously enough to take charge of what you do with the minutes and hours. Consider where you stand on matters of religious belief and practice, and do something about it, if called for. Make yourself a meaningful part of your community by serving in some way that benefits others. Read. Tune in to local artists and to time-honored greats. Get outside and enjoy all sorts of weather in every season of the year. Consider the vastness of the universe and your place in it. Life is short, and not to be wasted on matters that will soon enough cease to be of any concern.

49.

Rewrite Your Internal Script

You talk to yourself all the time, although you may not be aware of it. It's worth the effort to become aware, however, because you can have a profound influence, for better or worse, on your happiness and effectiveness. For example, you may have labeled yourself as a procrastinator. "I never do things until the last minute," you may tell yourself (and possibly others). Sure enough, the next time something arises that you could get started on in a timely fashion, you put it aside for "tomorrow." You already know that you'll postpone whatever it is, and so naturally, you do so. It is often the same in matters of food and weight. "The minute I lose a few pounds," you decide, "I always get a craving for chocolate." Lo and behold, you step on the scale and see a magic, missing three pounds. Now what was that...? Oh yes, chocolate!

Now let's just suppose that you were to change your internal script. Suppose, for example, that you ditched the "procrastinator" label. Instead, you said, "I always feel so much better when I do things as they occur to me. Then all of the worrying at the last minute is done away with." Instead of condemning yourself at the outset with a negative label, you nod your head and say, "I think I'll make that first phone call right now."

You can reprogram yourself regarding weight loss and eating, as well. You don't have to eat chocolate every time that you lose weight, even if that has been your pattern in the past. You can create new patterns, using the power of your own internal coaching. Next time that you step on the scale and see a loss, you can say: "Way to go! This deserves a treat. I'm going to put off cleaning the house and take a jog on this beautiful day."

The internal messages of failure and disappointment can easily turn into self-fulfilling prophecy, but so can the language of success and strength. Take the time to listen to yourself. Pinpoint the areas in which you give yourself a hard time. Dwell on what you want to be and do, and build that into a new script for yourself. The self-fulfilling prophecies will be a joy to behold.

50.

Learn to Deal with Gains

Weight gain happens to *everyone*. It's a sign that you're alive and in a constant state of change and growth. It's not to be dreaded or overemphasized. It's simply a fact of life. Yet it has a special power to disappoint and discourage us if we have to work to maintain a healthy weight. What matters, however, is not that weight gain happens; it's what we do about it.

Starving yourself is absolutely not the answer to weight gain. Studies have shown conclusively that your body has a physiological response to perceived starvation. Your body immediately, automatically, starts to conserve when it is denied adequate fuel. Translated, this means that when you try to crash your way through a weight-loss diet, your body is fighting you every step of the way.

Castigating yourself doesn't serve you, either. All that does is make you miserable with yourself, your life, and your daily intake of food. This is negative self-talk at its most destructive, because you're beating yourself up for something that happens naturally to everyone, and you're piling emotional baggage on your back at the very time when you want to be on top of your game.

If you're generally eating moderately and exercising regularly, you probably won't suddenly find yourself having grown several sizes larger. At any rate, it's helpful to respond early on when you see a gaining trend. Switching to an eating style that cuts back on fats and carbohydrates, and focuses on fresh vegetables and lean protein, will take off a quick gain. Eating big salads, fresh fruit, and moderate portions of poultry and fish reassures your body that you are not starving, while at the same time cutting out enough slow-metabolizing calories so that your body will have to burn stored fat.

If you add to that an internal cheerleading squad, you'll find that the response to weight gain is relatively painless. Don't say, "*Why* did you insist on eating that dessert last night? No one would have been offended. You're just an *idiot*." Instead say: "Oh, my. Look at that. The usual swing up. Time to turn the direction downward." You not only acknowledge the true state of affairs, you also affirm your ability and determination to keep leveling the balance as you go through the human body's normal ups and downs.

51.

Envision Change

The power of the human psyche is undeniable. People have the potential to overcome daunting odds, to rise to formidable challenges, and to make success stories of some of the worst conceivable situations. We survive shipwrecks, war, disabling accidents, and tragic losses. Many times, we do it with little or nothing more than the strength and determination of our own spirit.

Viewed in the context of life's most awe-inspiring challenges, the business of weight loss seems insignificant. Yet on a daily basis, it can demand a great deal of our energy and attention. When we're struggling without noticeable success, it can disappoint and depress us. One of the keys to moving beyond preoccupation and discouragement is envisioning a positive outcome.

It has been noted that top racecar drivers have a trick when their cars are headed for high-speed trouble. They don't look at the wall that they're hurtling toward, but rather at the path that they need to steer to escape an accident. Envisioning a positive outcome when you're on the weight-loss track is not that different.

You can begin by developing a habit of picturing yourself at your ideal weight. See yourself trim and healthy, fully engaged in life and wholesome activity. When you're entering one of those tailspin situations—the rich dessert is being served; the bowl of fatty chips is beckoning; the cheese plate is being passed for seconds or thirds—rather than fix your attention on the potential derailment of your goals, envision the path past it. Call on that habit of seeing yourself in your trim, ideal future. Sit up straighter, smile politely, shake your head with confidence, and say, "No, thanks. I've had enough."

52.

Make Short-Term Goals

Sometimes, the long haul seems just too long. It looks like a tunnel with no end in sight, and we become disheartened and unsure of our ability to stay the course. With no immediate gratification in sight, we're tempted to fall back on old habits that we find comforting. For someone struggling against excess weight, that may very well involve comfort food.

Depending on how much weight you want or need to lose, health-conscious weight loss can take time. A quick loss rarely stays off. It's the slow and steady reduction that will deliver long-term results. That makes short-term goals all the more helpful and important.

Key to successful short-term goal-setting is a realistic view. For example, you may be carrying an excess weight of thirty pounds. Realistically, healthy, moderate changes in eating and exercising habits will have you working toward your goal for several months. Some people may take a couple of years to lose that weight and consider it a job well done. In the meantime, you can make a short-term goal that focuses on behavior rather than what the scale says.

Concentrate on meeting a weekly goal of three or four one-hour aerobic sessions, or five hour-long brisk walks. Make it a goal to plan what and when you'll eat for a week. Consider your goal met when, at the end of the week, you've both planned and fulfilled the plan. Let these constructive patterns capture your attention, instead of the number of pounds that you lose each day or week.

When you set and reach short-term goals, you'll feel less compelled to step on the scale to chart your progress. You can wait a couple of weeks, or even a month, between weigh-ins, knowing that you're doing exactly what needs to be done to reach the long-term goals that you've set. When you see a slow and steady progress toward weight loss one month after another, you'll have the satisfaction of knowing that you're on the right track for *lasting* changes and good health.

53.

Rethink the Pantry

The first and most obvious solution to battling your temptations toward indulgent, undesirable foods is to remove them from your reach. Don't stock your refrigerator or pantry shelf with those items. Choose healthful, helpful alternatives. Or keep less food in the house, in general. If the temptation is not within reach, you're less likely to go to the trouble to give in to it.

It isn't always that easy, of course. If others in the house have different food requirements and preferences, you may find that the food there for someone else calls to your weakness. In that case, you may want to enlist the sympathy and support of housemates. Stock only small amounts of their favorite indulgences, and ask that they make a point of eating them when they are available instead of letting them sit there, dangling in front of your imagination like a lure. In fact, if they tend to let the goodies sit, they may not want or need them very much anyway. You needn't keep the stuff stocked. You can even ask them to enjoy their treats away from home, some or all of the time.

Sometimes, we use others as an excuse to keep our favorite treats around, even though we won't serve our weight-loss goals by eating them. The power of self-deception can be as strong as the power of positive thinking. Be ruthless in your assessment of your situation. Tell yourself the truth, and if the truth is painful, face it squarely, and strategize with courage. In the same way that you envision a positive outcome, you can create a constructive environment. Make the pantry your friend.

54.

Avoid Boredom Eating

Because food can be gratifying in an immediate sense, many people turn to eating when their imaginations let them down. They're engaged in a thankless chore, too tired to get busy with something meaningful, or simply at loose ends. To fight the "blahs," they trot along to the kitchen or snack shop and medicate themselves with food that they don't need. It may give them a quick lift, but it sure doesn't solve the problem.

Pay attention to boredom. Notice when it happens and what it's associated with. Do some soul searching about what's missing in your life on a higher level if you succumb to boredom with any regularity. If you're actually dealing with depression, think about getting help in dealing with that as the root cause for your ennui. Depression can have serious consequences for your health and long-term well-being. It is worthy of attention.

If you're bored because your life lacks interesting challenges, do something about it. Stop putting off that great adventure. Learn that new skill. Put some energy into deciding what really matters to you and how you can nurture it in more significant ways in your life. Opportunities abound for personal growth and change, but they aren't likely to hit you in the face. You have to go after them and make them happen. It's all about envisioning change. It's possible to defeat yourself before you ever start with a litany of "I can't," "The kids need me," or "I'm too tired." The reality is that you *can*, the kids need a parent who is alive and positive, and you won't be as tired if you're engaged in pursuits that inspire you.

If you're bored simply because you've become lazy, don't beat yourself up. Most of us have seasons when we lose our spark a little. Recognize that if you stay in that lazy, bored state, you're effectively wasting the days, hours, and minutes of the most precious gift that you will ever receive—your life. Get up off the sofa, put the chips away, and get busy doing something that means something to you. Eating because there's nothing better to do will become a thing of the past.

55.

Learn to Say No Without Guilt

Believe it or not, it's okay to say no when someone offers you food that you don't want to eat. People with health concerns do it all of the time, and often, they don't choose to explain. It's not rude for someone with diabetes to turn down a rich dessert. It's not offensive for someone with disastrously high cholesterol to take only a tiny portion of butter or an entrée made up of beef.

If you have determined that you need to lose weight for the sake of your health and well-being, you're dealing with a physical situation that warrants just as much care and attention as people who are dealing with health-threatening conditions of other sorts. You have the right, even the responsibility, to judge the wisdom of including something in your diet, even when you are a guest. Most hosts are well enough informed to realize that many people have to watch what they're eating for a variety of very sound reasons. You don't owe anyone an explanation. It's enough to say, "No, thanks." If your host seems to need more, you can simply say, "I never eat that. It doesn't agree with me." Enough said. You've been polite, and a polite host will accept it.

An alternative to the all-or-nothing approach, of course, is to ask for a tiny portion so that you can taste what your host has prepared or offered and give them the gratification of an admiring response. If, despite your request, you're served a full or large portion, go back to the trick of pushing aside all but the bite that you requested. If they insist that you have more, push the plate away with a smile and say, "I'd love to, but I really can't. That was certainly delicious!"

Guilt often drives us to work against what we know is best for us. Guilt almost always comes from the outside. It may be a historical guilt, based on a much-repeated message from parents or others in our childhood. Or it may be very present, offered by friends, colleagues, or family who have their own needs that they're trying to meet through us.

Remember that you are ultimately the one who is responsible for your welfare. Others will rarely put your well-being before concerns of their own. Taking care of yourself is not neglecting others. It's keeping yourself well and strong so that you can be a better, more compassionate friend, colleague, and family member.

56.

Expose the Myth of
Weight Loss as Happiness

Weight management has a significant role to play in good health and quality of life. Good health and an active life contribute meaningfully to a person's sense of optimism and energy. In these ways, weight loss may very well affect how happy a person feels.

People who have struggled with being overweight for any length of time, however, sometimes invest weight loss with the unrealistic expectations of a panacea, a magic path to "happily ever after." They develop a catch-all, "If only," that is tied directly to their success or failure to lose their extra weight. "If only" they weighed less, they would have more friends, they wouldn't feel depressed, they would get out more, they would finish their college education, they would have a better a job, a better mate, a better time. In other words, they would be happy.

It's all very well to keep the benefits of weight loss in mind when you need to lose weight. Doing so provides motivation and a positive vision of the future. Unfortunately, when you associate weight loss with happiness, you rob yourself of the joy that you could be experiencing right now. There's no question that the satisfaction of doing what you set out to do can add to your personal pleasure. Neither is it in doubt that feeling good about how you feel and look can give you a lift. But happiness doesn't reside in any one factor, and it doesn't come from the external. It comes from within an individual, and it can transcend the many ups, downs, ins, and outs of a lifetime.

Don't postpone your love of life and people. Don't wait to nurture an optimistic mindset that allows you grace in times of trouble and compassion in the midst of distress. If you need to lose weight, go for it. Look forward to the health and aesthetic benefits that you'll enjoy when you reach your goal. But understand that it is not the answer to life's challenges. You don't have to take off those pounds before you deal with other issues that may be weighing you down just as much. Weight loss is only one small piece of your day-to-day journey. Keep it in its place, and get on with the business of living life fully and meaningfully. If you do, happiness will follow.

57.

Choose Fresh over Preserved

Some of the most appealing characteristics of foods in their natural states are altered in preparation, and especially in preserving. Textures, smells, physical appearance, and flavor can all be changed to a remarkable extent. Open a can of green beans and compare the product to beans right off the vine if you have any doubts. This isn't to say that the canned beans can't be appetizing, but the preserved product is quite different from the unprocessed food from which it came.

There are advantages to including fresh rather than preserved foods in your diet. Fresh food contains the optimum amount of nutritional value. Good nutrition depends on a complex combination of vitamins, minerals, fiber, fats, proteins, water, and carbohydrates that occur in nature in delicate balance. Some nutrients only help us when they are ingested in tandem with other particular nutrients. Some components we need only in trace amounts, which is exactly how nature provides them in fresh food. Fiber content is invariably most present in foods that have not been manipulated.

When food is processed and preserved, nutrients can be substantially reduced or lost. Fiber is culled from a product as it is milled; heat and other processing components destroy delicate vitamins; and flavor and color are changed or lost. Of course, in order to make the finished product appealing to the buying public, manufacturers often introduce flavor additives, artificial colors, synthetic nutrients, and preservatives. Although all of this has to pass rigorous testing to determine its health safety, we don't really know what subtle differences it may make in how our bodies use it.

Fresh food also tends to take a little more work to eat, which is an advantage for anyone who tends to eat too much, too fast, or both. Raw fruits and vegetables contain a lot of water, which your body needs and which helps you feel full when you've eaten enough. They also require a lot of chewing, which can satisfy the "munchies" to which so many people fall prey. Fresh meat and dairy products are at their most nutritious and flavorful, and will satisfy the flavor yen in much more wholesome ways than processed foods with a lot of sauces, salt, sugar, or added fats.

Perhaps the greatest advantage to choosing fresh food as often as possible is the personal satisfaction that comes from knowing that you're doing something good for yourself. Fresh food is a treat, and the more of it you eat, the more you'll come to appreciate it over the processed stuff.

58.

Identify Empty Calories

The word "calorie" is used in its nutritional sense to measure the heat- or energy-producing value of food when oxidized by the human body. A given food is said to contain so many calories, by which we understand that it will take a certain amount of our body's energy to use that amount. If we take in fewer calories than we are burning, our bodies have to draw on stored calories in the form of fat. If we use up all of our stored fat, our bodies will start using muscle tissue as fuel. (This is not desirable. Among the muscles affected is your heart!) If our intake of calories exceeds what we burn, the excess is stored as fat. Therefore, if we eat more than we need, we gain fat weight.

Ideally, there's a marvelous efficiency to this system of fueling the human body. We take in nutrients and water by eating and drinking, and then our bodies oxidize the food, extracting the nutrients and putting them to work at their various jobs and eliminating the waste. We gain energy and thrive.

Weight-loss programs often focus on calories as a shorthand method of helping people do the math that accounts for weight loss: "X number of calories a day for a person of your gender, body type, activity level, and age will sustain your weight. X minus Y number of calories will cause you to lose weight." That's great as far as it goes. It works, if you keep track and are diligent.

In terms of sustaining the weight-loss effort and learning good habits for weight maintenance, however, the strict calorie calculus may not be the most effective or instructive. As long as you are using your allotted calories on nutritious, well-balanced consumption, all is well. But when you choose foods that offer little or no nutrition for some or most of that calorie intake, you do yourself a disservice. Foods lacking in nutritional value and overloaded with fat and sugar are what we call "empty" calories. They add up in terms of what your body can burn in a day, but they don't add to your body's nutritional needs. The net effect is that you still feel like you want to eat, even after you've used up your calorie allotment. Your body is still asking for the nutrition. It knows the difference.

Make a point of knowing the nutritional value of the foods that you eat. It should be obvious that a four-ounce potato offers far more nutrition than four ounces of potato chips, and contains none of the fat or salt. It's that sort of comparison that will help you identify and replace the empty calories in your diet. When you do, you'll feel more satisfied when you eat, you'll want to eat less, and you'll find it far easier to control your weight.

59.

Recognize the Binge Factors

You may be one of those people who wants a little taste of something forbidden once in a while to keep you feeling satisfied. And you may be able to take one bite of something over-the-top in calories and stop at that. However, many people suffering with extra weight find it a tricky or even risky proposition. One bite doesn't do it. Once started, they go for another bite, and another. One forbidden food leads to the next, and before they're done, they've consumed a month's worth of forbidden bites in a single half-hour.

This is binge eating, and for some people, it is a significant challenge to overcome. The effect of binge eating is more comprehensive than just slowing, stopping, or temporarily reversing the process of weight loss. It has a pronounced effect on self-image, optimism, perseverance, and physical well-being. It overloads your system for a time, and can set in motion a physical response that undermines your vitality. It easily becomes a bad habit that is remarkably difficult to break. At the heart of binge eating lies a temporary lack of connection with your intentions and goals.

People have found numerous ways of handling the binge factor. For some, the best solution is to be legalistic about when, where, and what they eat. They may develop a little list of "rules" that help them short-circuit the urge to binge. It can read something like this:

- Don't start. Then you won't have to stop.
- Never eat alone. It's too embarrassing to binge in front of someone else.
- Avoid food situations that include any friends or family members who make a habit of overeating. They'll only encourage behavior that you want to offset.
- Buy small quantities of tempting foods, or don't buy it at all.
- After one bite, put the food away and clean up immediately. Brush your teeth. Take a breather. It's harder to binge if you have to work to keep eating.

Rules have their place, and they may help you. Or you may look for a buddy whom you can call when you have the urge. Make yourself accountable, and talk it out instead of giving in.

60.

Plan Rewards for Meeting Goals

Life has more than enough hard spots in it, and often the highs seem few and far between. This is all the more reason why when you set a goal and reach it, you deserve to reward yourself. The reward gives you something to look forward to enjoying, and to look back on with pleasure.

In the interest of sustaining your successful forward motion, it's important to think about what you will offer yourself as a reward. Many people who have struggled with weight control and overeating have a history of rewarding themselves with food. This has some obvious drawbacks for someone who is celebrating a weight-loss achievement.

When you take control of issues relating to weight management, you make a strong move toward loving and caring for yourself. So why not make that the criterion for the rewards that you give yourself along the way? Mini-rewards may include a day at the beach or hiking, an afternoon at a museum or a favorite spa, a new golf club, a garment that you couldn't have worn before, or even a big bouquet of fresh-cut flowers. A day away from responsibilities—a personal day from the office or childcare—can be a great treat. If your chosen reward gives you pleasure or satisfaction, if it feeds your spirit and your sense of accomplishment, then it meets the general criterion of caring for yourself.

When the benchmark is a big one, a larger reward may be in order. Maybe you can plan for the half-year mark with a week away. Perhaps you've wanted to get involved in a new hobby, enhance your professional skills, or join a community effort of some kind. While none of these activities needs to wait for an excuse, we often put off such things for lack of pretext. Let your success in meeting a goal be a good reason, and enjoy it fully.

The motivations for losing weight often come laden with bad news or negative feelings. The doctor says that you've got to do it to preserve your health. The mirror tells you that you don't look the way that you want to look. Your joints remind you that you're carrying a larger body around than you were designed to carry.

Allow yourself something positive. Hold out the promise of a gift that you'll enjoy and benefit from. When you reach your goal, fulfill the promise to yourself. The more practice you have at treating yourself well in all respects, the more automatic those helpful rewards will become. Keep in mind that you're worth it, and enjoy.

61.

Make Friends with Mirrors

Preoccupation with appearance is one of the most pervasive traps in modern society, and it can rob of us of joy in life and pleasure in who and what we are. The image that we see of ourselves in the mirror is almost never the objective view that we think it is. Almost everyone has particular features of face and body that they consider flaws or weaknesses. It might be the size of your nose or hips; it might be the cut of your chin or waist. Whatever it is, it looms large in your own vision. It's the first thing that you notice and the most important thing on your list of physical traits.

On the other hand, you probably also have features that you're quite proud of. You may check to make sure that they're still there and that you still consider them pleasing. Of course, the day invariably comes when they do change. That's the nature of living and aging.

The problem with this preoccupation is that people overemphasize how they look, and neglect their other qualities. Appearance may or may not reflect character. Neither does it tell the whole story of your temperament—your cheerfulness, industry, energy, or stamina—or your intellect. In the grand scheme of things, and certainly over the course of your lifetime, those aspects of who and what you are that are not tied to your appearance are the ones that ripen and improve. Those are the things that earn self-respect and the respect of others. Those are the things that help us relate in meaningful, loving ways to others and make a difference in the world.

How often do you look in a mirror in a day? Check it out. Don't change your regular routine, but take note of when, where, and why you stop to look. Pay attention to what you check first when you look at yourself. Then consider how important that is in relation to who you are. The mirror doesn't need to be your daily judge and jury. It only reveals the *surface* of you, and it does that imperfectly because you are not an objective viewer. Go ahead and let the mirror serve the purpose of showing you that your hair is straight, your face is clean, and your clothes aren't on backward. Then leave it alone for the day. You have better things to do with your self-esteem.

62.

Focus on Your Successes

It's easy to place emphasis on our failures. Often, as we grow up, we hear a lot more feedback about what's wrong with our behavior or performance than what is right. Our parents had the difficult job of teaching us to be responsible, caring adults, and to do that, they disciplined us when we headed in the wrong direction. In school, our performance was graded, and many of us developed sensitivity toward our failure to excel perfectly. The system was designed to make us achievers, and achievers don't typically deal well with less-than-sterling achievement.

Weight loss is rarely a linear process, with one success following another. You will often hit plateaus or setbacks when you set your path to lose. But focusing on the times and ways that you "fail"—that is, when you stop losing or regain a few pounds—will not help you get back on track. There may be some educational value in the so-called failures, and if you treat them that way, you may find better strategies for weight loss in the future. But you may also sabotage your potential for future success. Discouragement and self-loathing will replace determination and self-respect.

Rather than fill your thoughts with ways that you have failed, in the short run, to do what you set out to do, fix your attention on the ways in which you have succeeded. Consider any factors that may have played a role in your success. Place your successes firmly in your vision for what you will do next. Build strategies on what you've done right, and draw energy from the knowledge that it was you who did it.

63.

Plan Your Snacks

You probably know what time of day you typically want a snack. Many people find that the stretch between lunch and dinner is a long haul, and they want a little something to munch on in the midafternoon. Others crave a morsel midmorning. Still others find that a bite of something before bed helps them relax and fall asleep. Whatever your pattern is, plan ahead so that you're sure to have wholesome snacks available when and where you need them.

Start by purchasing your planned snacks ahead of time. We run into trouble when we wait until the urge to eat strikes before we forage. In a hungry mood, we're more likely to give in to whim and convenience, which can lead to choices that don't serve our best interests. As with food at regular meals, choose items that are low in fat and sugar and high in nutrition. Crunchy, chewy fresh vegetables and fruit take more time to eat and satisfy the chewing urge. High-protein foods stay with you longer.

Next, when you bring your snack supplies home, think about prepackaging measured amounts that are ready to go when you are. A reasonable amount of food for a snack has to be measured against what else you are consuming throughout the day. If you're involved in planned weight loss, you've probably got some guidelines about total consumption based on calories or number of servings of certain food groups. Snacks need to be added into the total if such a plan is going to work.

If you measure the food out in snack- or sandwich-sized plastic containers at a time that you aren't hungry for it, you'll probably find it easier to be honest about how much you give yourself than if you grab the food when you're hungry. Premeasuring may not ensure that you won't eat more, but at least it gives you an accurate signal when you've eaten enough. It will take a conscious decision to overeat.

Make a point of having a big glass of water or cup of tea before you snack. You may feel hungry simply because you're dehydrated. Fluid will also help fill you up so that you don't feel like eating as much.

Whatever fits your particular schedule and needs, plan ahead, and plan for success. Snacking doesn't have to interfere with weight management. It just takes planning.

64.

Put Food on the Back Burner

When you focus on food, even in the interest of maintaining a healthful way of eating, it can sometimes backfire. Constant attention to food keeps food and its consumption at the forefront of your thinking, which can lead to overindulgence. That is *not* in the interest of maintaining a wholesome way of eating.

Find times where food is not allowed to be in your thoughts. When you do have to eat, make sure that you have something simple, and avoid preparing time-consuming meals. It can be helpful to plan a lean day a week. Choose meals comprised of raw fruit and vegetables, soup, whole-grain bread and cereal, and fish or poultry that can be cooked lightly and quickly or ahead of time. The idea is to stop thinking and planning about food for the day, and to spend as little time in the kitchen as possible. Some people, after trying this for a while, enjoy it so much that they make it more the rule than the exception, saving elaborate meals for once or twice a week and special occasions. They literally put food on the back burner.

Another way of making food less of a daily preoccupation is to plan at least one carryover meal a week that you prepare when you have the time—maybe on the weekend or a quiet evening. If you make enough of a homemade soup for several meals, for example, there is very little preparation and forethought needed on the days when you eat the leftovers. Roasting a turkey or turkey breast provides enough to be sliced and warmed for a number of meals. A big pot of vegetarian chili goes a long way, as does a double batch of low-fat fish cakes. Choose your favorite standards, and make enough to put aside for another meal.

It can help, as well, to prepare an abundance of fixings for salad at one time. If you store the non-leafy ingredients in good plastic containers and put washed and dried greens in bags with paper towels to absorb any excess moisture, the food will keep for almost a week, and you can prepare salad with virtually no thought or time at all.

The point is to take your mind off food more often. You can continue to eat well without obsessing on the subject. The more you take your focus off food, the more natural it will become, and the more time you'll find for other pursuits. The effort will yield both a better-rounded life and a less round physique.

65.

Practice Graceful Ways to Say No

One of the greatest life skills you will learn is the ability to say no with grace. It comes up all the time: declining requests for donations; turning away unwanted suitors; guiding your children away from disaster; resisting sales pitches; or taking your eating habits into your own hands. If you can learn to make your decision based on good judgment from within instead of pressure from without—and do it in a way that allows you self-respect and dignity—you will be far ahead of the pack.

Planting several truths securely in your mind will help. First, no one is indispensable. A negative response from you is not, ultimately, going to ruin anyone's life, leave them permanently in the lurch, or mortally offend them. If they want something from you that you decide not to give them, will they be disappointed? Probably. Will they live? Absolutely. Will they get over it? If they don't, you're dealing with someone who needs to grow up.

Second, unless you have already promised to say yes, there is no reason why you can't say no. In giving an honest answer to whatever is proffered, you've done your part by taking responsibility for yourself. It is a kindness to both you and the person you're dealing with. Getting over the negative consequences of caving in to decisions that you know are not good for you is far more devastating than being conscientiously honest in the first place.

Third, even a yes can be turned into a no if you think better of a decision that you've made. You should never feel obliged to hold yourself to a promise that on reflection you realize should not have been made. It may require you to eat some crow. You may feel embarrassed or cause some inconvenience or even pain. But the damage will be far less than it would be if you insisted on following through on an ill-advised commitment.

So where does grace fit into the equation? Grace resides in seeking to understand and appreciate the other person's point of view while still saying no for yourself. It is being true to yourself and disappointing another with compassion and honesty. Inner peace ensues because you know that you have made the wisest decision and stuck with it.

This may sound a little heavy when you put it in the context of eating or not eating food that someone offers you. However, many of the relatively minor decisions that we make from day to day become far easier when we already know our mindset on the big-picture issues. You can say no with grace to food that you do not want or need.

66.

Redefine Sexiness

Despite the current obsession with celebrity and glamour, sexiness does not reside in the size or shape of your body. Many a healthy, attractive person—well within the advisable weight range for gender, age, and body type—has undertaken punishing weight-loss regimes in the interest of looking and feeling sexier to a romantic partner.

If you have ever entertained the notion that you can only be sexy if you lose those last ten pounds, think again. Sexiness is never in the packaging. It's in your attitudes. Can you make yourself more attractive by paying attention to grooming and style? Of course you can. But if you think that losing weight is the ultimate answer to becoming beautiful, think again.

The business of attraction between romantic partners is a subtle and complicated one. It involves a basic chemistry, predispositions to certain characteristics in a partner, and sympathy of spirit. At its best, it is built on solid respect, friendship, compassion, and mutual support. No lack of body fat can replace such components. Being thinner will never make a good substitute for being romantic, demonstrative, playful, and connected.

If you are dealing with a partner who makes your weight an issue in terms of romance and intimacy, take a second look at who you are with and why. The shape of your body is superficial. The beauty and sexiness of your personality, attitudes, and behavior are what count.

There are many very good reasons for losing weight. That it will make you irresistibly sexy isn't one of them.

67.

Make Variety a Priority

Nothing kills a weight-loss plan—no matter how effective—faster than the tedium of eating the same few foods day after day. Boredom is not a particularly productive state for most people. You may quickly find yourself discouraged and sneaking treats to break free of the ennui. Or you may wake up one morning and face the same weight-loss breakfast that you've endured for a month and say, "Forget it! I can no longer do this every day!" The next thing that you know, you're back to old habits.

In addition, a limited choice of foods for any length of time may actually deprive you of nutrients that you need. You may be hitting the high spots nutritionally, but neglecting trace elements that help you metabolize and use the food that you eat. One possible outcome, in this case, is that you'll begin to crave foods inconsistent with weight loss that contain those trace elements. Once you give in to the cravings, you may find your dietary plan permanently subverted.

Perhaps the most problematic outcome of a limited range of food in your weight-loss plan is that it does nothing to help you build better eating habits on the other side of weight loss. Unless you learn how to maintain a healthy diet that also maintains your target weight, you'll be on the gain-lose-gain treadmill for a lifetime.

A growing number of weight-loss programs have been built on the understanding that variety is important. These programs suggest categories of food, with lists of options in each category and a master plan for how many servings of each category you can consume in a day. The great advantage of this approach is that a broad range of foods can remain a part of your plan. It allows for a good measure of personal choice and gives you a healthy mix of nutritional sources. Such a plan is so user-friendly that it also serves as a viable tutorial for maintenance once you've reached your target weight.

68.

Know the Dangers of Excess

When you want to lose weight, it's natural to want it over and done with as quickly as possible. Being at your target weight is so much more appealing than what it takes to get there. But there is no natural or healthy way to rush weight loss. The two most effective means for shedding extra pounds—reduced consumption of food, and exercise—offer the best and longest-lasting results when you put them to use in moderation. When you take either or both to extremes, you set yourself up for some counterproductive or even potentially dangerous side effects.

Studies have shown, for example, that when you skip meals, you can actually slow your metabolic rate, and thus burn fewer calories. Eating regularly, spreading nutrition and calories throughout the day, gives your system a steady flow of energy and nutrients and keeps it operating efficiently. There has also been research that documents a strong correlation between strenuous dieting and the onset of eating disorders. Eating a balanced diet that includes plenty of fiber, cuts back on fats and refined sugars, and is spread out through the day will offer the best, most natural way to trim down without risk.

Regular exercise has been shown to offer many health benefits, but the high visibility of amateur and professional athletes who often train and perform at extreme levels, as well as our "more is better" mentality, make it easy to see why people today might be prone to exercise excess. Like overzealous dieting, an excess of exercise poses real threats to your health and well-being. Too much vigorous exercise has been implicated in sudden heart attacks in people at risk; joint, tendon, ligament, and muscle injuries to the lower body for people carrying extra weight; depressed immune systems; hormonal imbalances; and even eating disorders.

However, *moderate* exercise contributes positively to stress reduction, calorie burning, muscle building, and weight loss. It is also sustainable and much less likely to lead to injury. Despite what you might expect, it is probably more effective than excessive exercise in the long run.

69.

Be Realistic at Family Gatherings

Family gatherings can be wonderful occasions full of nurturing, love, and shared history. But they can also be a challenge, especially for people who have fought the battle of the bulge for most of their lives. When we gather with family, we bring the past along with us. Old self-images rear their sometimes-ugly heads, and we find ourselves reverting to old habits. While the get-together can be a wonderful event, it can also bear resemblance to walking in a minefield.

One obvious difficulty that often arises for someone working on weight management is the issue of the family's eating style versus the individual's. Ideas about eating change from one generation to the next, and if your family's philosophy of eating doesn't compare to yours, you can easily find yourself with a plateful of food that you'd rather not eat. If a member of your extended family has made the food, it can be remarkably difficult to say, "No, thank you." You may even be offered a plate of what used to be your favorite food. Then you have to deal with the added pressure of refusing something that was made "just for you."

The food itself may not be the crux of your challenge, however. For many, the psychological exchanges that occur among family members at such gatherings can be as hard as or harder than the food offered. A sibling may have you pegged as an overeater; a cousin may remember the days when you had dimples on your elbows from excess weight; a parent may have negative opinions about your life decisions. As the past surfaces within the group, you may find yourself slipping into old coping patterns that no longer reflect who you are or what you want from life.

Chances are that you know what happens when the family gathers, because you've experienced it many times before. That knowledge can give you a powerful tool for coping in positive ways with the situation and your own feelings about it. Plan ahead for what you will do about food and drink. Think it through before you arrive. Make adjustments that take into account the relatively short time that such a gathering is likely to last. Carry with you a solid image of the person that you are becoming and want to be—then *be* that person.

70.

Visualize Future Success

While spending your time in the past or the future to the neglect of today seems a sorry waste of the life you've been given, it should be said that reflection on the past can be instructive if you have a will to learn from past mistakes and successes. And anticipation of the future can help you fulfill your fondest dreams by providing a strong vision of what you want and how you might go about getting it.

Sometimes, you can set our own limits with a lack of vision or imagination. You can choose instead to expand your horizons and make the most of all that you have and are. You can "see" your future and then bring it about by taking steady, regular steps in the direction that you've chosen. If you've been frustrated in the past, examine what went awry and consider the part that you played in it. With that understanding, you can strategize for new and better ways to reach your goals and gather the energy to actively pursue them.

Consider now what you're aiming for. If you're on the way to reaching your target weight, develop a strong vision of how you will sustain the effort required, and what reaching your goal will produce in your energy level, quality of life, and appearance. But don't stop there. Make room for a much grander vision. Include what you want to do with your talents, where you want to be in your experience or career, where you want to be geographically, what you expect or hope to accomplish, and what you want to contribute to others and the world around you. Try writing it down; even if it's a single paragraph, putting it into words may be just the motivating exercise that you need to move forward. Success imagined is often the first step toward success realized.

71.

Focus on Your Appearance Assets

What do you see first when you look in the mirror? If you're like most people, your attention jumps instantly to whatever it is that you see as your physical flaws. Your right eye is a little higher than your left. You see the shadow of a double chin. Your stomach has more cushion than you like. Your nose is too big. And so on.

Nearly everyone has at one time or another identified features or aspects of their appearance that are less than ideal. In many cases, they see something that with a bit of effort could be changed. In others, they're dealing with things that were written into their genes. Focusing on these so-called "imperfections" can have a negative effect on your self-image that far outweighs their importance, and can prevent you from developing a well-balanced view of yourself.

Take an inventory of your physical traits. For every negative characteristic that you observe, find at least one positive. Keep a list as you go, with negatives in a column on the left and positives in a column on the right. When you've completed the list or filled a page, take the paper and tear it down the middle lengthwise so that the two lists are now on separate pages. Then take the negative page, ball it up in a wad, and toss it in the wastebasket. Take the positive page and put it somewhere convenient that allows you to readily refer to it. When negative thoughts about yourself arise, return to it.

It is easy to dwell on what bothers you about your appearance, but it takes an effort to focus special attention on your assets. The more you do it, though, the more realistic your vision of yourself will become. Over time, you may begin to notice more that you like about yourself that doesn't depend at all on appearance. When that really takes hold, you will be able to put appearance, weight, and the idiosyncrasies that make you you into perspective.

72.

Allow Plateaus

Everything living experiences seasons. When life is new and young, there is a season of vigorous growth. As age advances, growth slows, and size often stabilizes. There are seasons of rest, seasons of reproduction, and seasons of bloom, ebbs and flows, quiet and excitement.

It's in the nature of your own physical existence that you, too, experience seasons. Think back over your years, and characterize the different times of your life. Remember the days of growth spurts and the times when you thought you would never grow another inch. Think of instances when you were on the learning curve, struggling to master a skill or a concept—then something connected, and what had been difficult finally became understandable.

The natural pace of life and change can sometimes make us impatient. We see where we want to be and it doesn't happen *now*. Yet nature has its own logic. Often, we can't see the process that goes on. That doesn't change the fact that it does, indeed, go on.

Losing weight and shaping up in a healthful way take time. In the midst of losing weight or gaining strength, we often hit times when progress seems to slow or stop. We go from impatience to discouragement to despair. Then, suddenly, another spurt of progress occurs. But only if in the midst of the plateau, we continue to do what's needed. Weight loss does not occur on a schedule. A great many factors are at work in the human body at any given time, and we add some new factors when we set in motion the business of burning stored fat and changing our metabolic rate. The pace at which we see results may vary, but that doesn't mean that the results are no longer in the works.

Once you realize that plateaus and slowdowns are all part of the process, you can learn to stick with your resolve even in the midst of them. Think of them as breathers—necessary pauses in the body's action—and keep doing what you're doing.

73.

Measure Your Servings

Do you know how much you eat? Maybe you do, and maybe you don't. It's amazing how many people struggle with weight loss for years, convinced that they don't eat a lot. Yet the weight stays on or actually increases over time.

Sometimes, people nosh their way through the day in a distracted state and don't pay attention to the fact that they're eating. More often, they know what they eat, and they know how many servings they have of what they eat. The problem is their notion of what counts as a serving.

When doctors and other experts spell out guidelines for weight loss, they usually create a plan that recommends a certain number of servings of any food or food group. To know what they mean by the word "serving," you have to read through the particular guidelines that you're following. The side panel on a cereal box routinely reports nutrition information according to one serving. But one kind of cereal considers one serving to be one cup of the cereal, while another, higher-fat, sugary cereal may specify one quarter-cup. In the case of the cereal manufacturers, they understand that the buying public expects one serving of any cereal (regardless of its makeup) to contain approximately the same number calories as the rest. So the people who make and sell cereal simply adjust the volume of the cereal that they call one serving.

On some diet programs, one serving is actually one unit of the food. One serving of strawberries might be one-quarter of a cup, and you'd be allowed two servings of the berries in a single sitting. One serving of beef might be designated as one ounce, which means that at a single sitting, you would be allowed four servings. A more common understanding of "serving" would be the standard total of that particular food for one meal. Thus, one serving of strawberries would be a half-cup, while one serving of beef would be four ounces.

Having said all that, and even knowing all that, some people still don't know how much they eat. They don't actually measure a cup. They eyeball it. Or they measured once, and now they're gauging by what they remember about how it looked in a certain dish.

The only accurate way to know how much you're eating is to measure it. If you think that you're consuming one designated serving and routinely, it turns out to be twice that, you can see how you might quickly find the weight staying on or moving upward. It only takes a moment to measure food, which is far less than it takes to lose a pound of extra weight. Measuring cups and a simple food scale are all it will take to get in touch with the amounts of your food consumption.

74.

Uncover Food Associations

You may not have a well-defined memory of what foods you associate with joy, but scents, sounds, and situations can often trigger comforting memories of a happy moment in your past, when food played a part in your sense of being loved and happy. It's natural to want to relive the moment, even if it's only by eating a few cookies.

If a cookie will enhance the moment of nostalgia, maybe that's just what you need. In terms of weight management, you also need to know what it is that you're really after when the urge to eat the cookie strikes. It helps you put it in perspective, for one thing, and recognize that the cookie can't really make you happy. The source of the good feelings is not the food, but rather a loving moment from your past.

You'll be better served by focusing your attention on fostering your most important relationships so that such moments continue in your present and future than by concentrating on the foods associated with them. One last reminder: A single bite of that cookie will leave you with just as much flavored memory as a half-dozen bites will.

75.

Plan Ahead for Social Situations

Most social events include food and drink of some kind as part of the entertainment. If you're in the midst of a weight-loss regime, you'll want to consider what offered foods will keep you on the path toward your goals, as well as touching your sense of enjoyment. If you're maintaining a preferred weight, you'll want to consider how an event fits in with your overall strategy and take steps to control eating and drinking.

Remember, first of all, that alcoholic drinks are quite costly, in terms of calorie intake. Moderate levels of alcohol won't undo you and your weight-control efforts, though they will slow you down, but heavy drinking most assuredly will cause problems. Such drinking will also pose significant health risks if you don't have it under control. It can be helpful and refreshing to intersperse a glass of water or seltzer between any alcoholic beverages. Because alcohol dehydrates you, the water will replenish your system. It will also offset drinking more alcohol in a vain attempt to quench your thirst.

Remember, too, that party food often includes offerings that are not over-the-top in fat, sugar, and calorie content. One of the pluses in this age of health-consciousness is the increased awareness of people's desire to have healthy alternatives to rich and fattening foods. You can keep the intake of the fattening choices under control, even at a party. Go ahead and taste the richest offerings, but to satisfy your hunger, feast on the salads, raw vegetables, and lower-fat protein sources. You'll leave the party satisfied on both the hunger and the moderation fronts.

Social gatherings focus, by definition, on people getting together. These events are opportunities to enjoy the companionship of others. The food is a pretext or a scene-setter, by and large; it's not the point. At least, it doesn't have to be the point *for you*. Focus on your friends, family, or colleagues on such social occasions. Let the food and drink be the background and the people be the foreground of your social life.

76.

Be Your Own Reference Point

No one walks in your shoes but you. Yet when social pressures bear down on us, this reality has an unfortunate tendency to slip out of our conscious thoughts and leave us vulnerable. We want to please others. We want their approval and moral support. We want to be like them so that they'll like us and want to be with us.

We may also want to be relieved of the burden of responsibility inherent in thinking and deciding for ourselves. If a friend of yours is a workout enthusiast, you may think, "Maybe I should be doing that, too. She sure looks good." Maybe another loves to dine out, constantly enjoying food and drink with fun-loving impunity. You think, "Maybe I should follow his lead. Everyone adores him."

The thing is that you aren't your friends. You're you. Only you can discern what will make your life meaningful and satisfying to you. You may entertain passing thoughts that pleasing everyone around you, or being like them, is the path to that meaningful, satisfying life. However, at the moments when your common sense kicks in, you realize that it isn't so.

In truth, you can't please everyone. What makes one person in your life happy is guaranteed to bother someone else. Rather than spend your time and energy deciding whom you'll concentrate your people-pleasing efforts on, concentrate on pleasing yourself. You may be surprised to discover that people do not love you less when you choose to be yourself and do what satisfies you. At the same time, with practice, you'll discover the true meaning and benefits of integrity. The essence of integrity has to do with being complete and undivided. When you know yourself and are true to yourself, you have integrity. There is little in life that offers more meaning or satisfaction than that.

When you suffer the temptation to let other people be your reference point, think about all they do not and cannot know or understand about what makes you who and what you are. Neither will they ultimately take responsibility for your decisions or the course of your life. That's up to you. Give yourself the time to get to know your own mind and heart. Live your life in accordance with that knowledge. Have the courage to be your own reference point.

77.

Remember Water

Water is arguably the most important substance that you ingest. Two-thirds of your body's composition is water. Water is the primary medium by which nutrients are transported through your body. It plays a major role in nearly every process of your body. It is also a must for the building that your body does daily to replace cells, create new tissue, and heal. It helps maintain your body temperature, and it carries waste and toxins out of your system.

The good news is that most of the food that you eat contains water. Even when you don't remember to drink a glass of water, you're taking it in through the food that you eat. In fact, the purest water that you're likely to find is contained in the fruits and vegetables that you eat.

The challenging news is that while the average adult body contains approximately forty-five quarts of water, it loses about three quarts daily through various sorts of excretion. (This can fluctuate widely, depending on your activity level and the climate in which you live. In the desert, you could lose closer to ten quarts daily.) The balance of water needs to be maintained for all of the vital work that your body does to keep you alive and well. That means drinking as much as eight eight-ounce glasses of water a day. Remember that water is not the same as fluid. Drinks that contain sugar, caffeine, or alcohol are not good options to satisfy your water needs. They contain ingredients that offset the effect that food and exercise has on your system.

When you drink water, you help your body operate efficiently. You offset the sensation of hunger that may sometimes actually be unrecognized thirst. You also satisfy the emotional need to put something in your mouth. So drink up.

78.

Seek a Doctor's Advice

If you're thinking about or involved in a weight-loss effort, make sure that you involve your medical doctor along the way. Taking off a significant amount of weight should involve a medical consultation.

How you lose, how much you lose, and how quickly you lose should be discussed with your health professional in the context of your overall health history. Genetic and lifestyle factors need to be kept in mind, as does your present health profile. Your doctor has a history of your particular body, and is better equipped than the average lay person to assess risk factors.

There's a lot of false information that makes the rounds among quasi-qualified health gurus. Health, fitness, and weight control are big business these days, and there's a lot of fine print in their advertising that you may not bother to read. The surest sign that you're dealing with a responsible counselor on the subject of weight loss and weight control is the caveat that you keep your doctor in the loop.

79.

What You're Teaching Your Children

Your weight-related habits and attitudes have a profound effect on your general health and well-being. If you have a family with children at home, your habits also have a profound effect on their attitudes and the habits that they learn.

Keep several factors in mind. First, if you are always preoccupied with matters of weight and food, your children are likely to follow suit. Without your ever addressing the subject directly to them, they'll pick up your anxieties and internalize them. By the time they are adolescents, the fact that you make such a big deal about weight will be added to societal and peer pressure and make weight a very big deal to them, as well. Unfortunately, such emphasis can be implicated in the development of poor self-image and eating disorders.

Your preoccupation with weight teaches them a set of values that you may not intend. Any ongoing focus on weight inevitably translates into a preoccupation with appearances. At the most critical period of their emotional and psychological development, young people who invest most of their attention in how they look stand to lose an appreciation for their more lasting potential and traits, such as perseverance, loyalty, honesty, compassion, kindness, or strength of purpose.

Children may also pick up the ways in which you criticize yourself and learn to criticize themselves in a similar way. Instead of focusing and building on their strengths, they may learn to judge themselves harshly and lose that marvelous ability to live with optimism and energy that is inherent in youth. In addition, they may feel judged by you. If you feel strongly about your own weight issues, after all, why wouldn't you feel that strongly about theirs?

If you suspect that your own issues with weight, diet, or fitness may have already been passed along to your kids, don't despair. One of the most meaningful ways in which you as a parent can model growth and maturity is to talk freely and show by your actions the ways in which your own understanding and behavior is changing and developing. As you gain perspective about how your weight concerns fit with the rest of life and relationships, your kids can grow with you. Don't hide your struggles from them. Let them see you struggle and overcome. If you do, you'll be well on the way to raising a new generation of people who can overcome problems, as well.

80.

Find Likeminded Support

If you have resolved to deal with the weight issues in your life, you know that you have challenges to face and overcome. It can be a lonely and discouraging process at times. You can lose your resolve and confidence. You can tire of the effort and be tempted to give up. You can overreact to setbacks and lose your belief in your own power to change. You can get lost in your own complicated psyche and find it difficult to keep your perspective and hope.

Having a partner to plan and work with can make an enormous difference in how you feel and how you do. There are plenty of people who want to resolve the constant battle with weight concerns. Just like you, they want to develop a life strategy that allows them to reach and maintain a healthy weight and then stop worrying about it all the time.

When you partner with another person or group of people, you have the combined resources of all of the people involved. When your resolve is slipping, call on a companion to revive your spirits. You can hold yourself accountable by being accountable to another person or group. This can be especially meaningful if you have a history of false starts. A spotty track record can undermine your confidence in successfully fulfilling your intentions. When someone else knows what you intend and wants regularly to hear about how you're doing, you have added motivation that can help build a new self-image and keep you on track.

There's an added value to sharing your progress toward a healthy weight and more productive attitude. You not only receive help, you give it. Any teacher will tell you that it's the teacher who learns the most. As you encourage another person in his or her efforts, you are encouraging yourself. You are giving yourself the same pep talks, finding the same insights, and learning the same strategies that you promote in the other person. It reinforces what you know, and may challenge you to find new ways to understand and express what you are learning.

You may have a close friend who is also getting control of his or her weight and would like a partner in the effort. Or you may want to find a group which focuses on the issue. In either case, if you've struggled unsuccessfully in the past, you can have renewed hope in the future. We are put on this planet in the company of other human beings. We're designed to be in relationships. The companionship and camaraderie of human society doesn't only work in the good times. It works in the challenging times. You don't have to do it alone.

81.

Take Aging into Account

Your body changes as you age. Your skin and hair become drier and less supple. Your joints stiffen up. The ratio of muscle to fat shifts—we tend to gain fat with age—and the fat itself tends to redistribute so that your shape alters. These changes happen gradually and naturally. They happen at various rates to different people, depending on each person's health, lifestyle, and genetic tendencies. You will experience age-related physical changes at every stage of your life, some of which have a direct effect on your weight and the ease with which you control it. You will be able to affect some of the changes or the rate at which they happen. Others you will have no control over.

It helps to be clear about the aging effects that you can do something about—versus the ones that you can't. Some changes are best accepted with grace and compensated for with positive changes on other fronts. On the other hand, some individuals shrug their shoulders too soon and too often about the ways that their bodies are changing. "I can't stop the aging process," they say, and allow themselves to weaken and gain weight with the passing years.

While it's true that your body will look different over time, it is not true that you have to let what you do for your health slip away. Granted, it may take more time and effort to achieve the sorts of results you could achieve at a younger age, but you can still keep the weight down and the strength up. The more consistently you exercise and pay attention to what, how, and when you eat, the better able you will be to manage your weight and maintain muscle mass.

It's good to keep in mind, at the same time, that research has suggested that a little extra fat as you age may actually be to your health advantage. At an older age, the higher end of the healthy weight range may be more realistic and better for you than the lower. Exercise requirements and strictures are also likely to change over time. Some of the things you used to do for exercise may need to be replaced with routines that are better suited to your present conditions.

Your doctor can and should advise you, but you will also be able to gauge yourself by the way that you feel. Don't expect to do everything that you've done in the past into the indefinite future. You can get equal or more benefit from a variety of exercise options. Neither should you expect the dimensions and average weight of your youth to continue as you enter middle age and older. Let your new chapters write themselves in reference to the present, instead of pinning your expectations to the past.

82.

Take It Easy

Issues regarding your weight are one small part of your life. You are more than what you weigh, and your life is more than how you look.

In the midst of weight-management efforts, keep your perspective. Give plenty of time and attention to your relationships. The people in your life, after all, are probably the most important part of your happiness and daily activity. Nurture the important relationships in your life. Enjoy every moment of them. Reach out to others and make them part of what is deepest and richest in your life.

Pay due attention to your work. Whether it's a vocation, a hobby, or a job, it is part of the way that you make a meaningful contribution to your family, your community, and society at large. It is a worthy effort, deserving of pride and interest. Give it your best, and make the most of it.

Remember to tend to the needs of your spirit. Life presents us with more than enough questions. It's up to each of us to invest some time in searching for answers that will guide us through the hard times, motivate us in the good times, and anchor our lives to something bigger than ourselves. Your religious beliefs need feeding and honing, your intellectual life needs challenging, and your perspective on the world requires input on a regular basis. Carve out time for matters of the spirit. It will pay dividends in peace and perspective.

Most of all, love the gift of life that you've been given. You will experience troubles. Everyone does. But you also have the hope of joy, love, and wonderful moments in time. Don't let your worries get you down. Take it easy, and enjoy the gifts.

83.

Develop Positive Self-Talk

You are probably your own harshest critic. You make value judgments constantly about who you are, what you do, and how you look. Those judgments turn into a daily dialogue within oneself. Many times they turn into a litany of negative feedback.

Keep a notebook with you for a week or so, with the intention of recording what you say to yourself. If you drop a glass in the sink and it shatters, make a note of your internal response. You may level sarcasm at yourself with a comment like, "That was *really* bright." If you drip gravy down the front of your shirt, pay attention to the self-addressed editorial, "What a slob I am!"

The point is that you talk to yourself all of the time. The extent to which your self-talk is negative is the extent to which you do yourself a disservice. Negativity saps your energy and robs you of joy. It defeats you before you try, and leaves you blue. In the arena of weight loss, it skews your view of yourself and makes the issue of weight more important than it ought to be.

You don't have to settle for negative self-talk. The benefit of paying attention to it and writing it down is that you can learn to redirect it. Instead of castigating yourself for an accident, you can say, "Oops. I'm human, after all." Instead of denigrating your abilities, you can say, "That was a good effort, but there's more to learn. What did I do right? What can I improve?" Instead of judging your appearance negatively, find your most attractive physical attributes and flaunt them, not only to others, but also to yourself.

If you can be your own worst critic, you can also learn to be your own strongest advocate and cheerleader. There's nothing pompous or conceited about knowing your positive attributes and consciously appreciating them. You know how often your heart is in the right place. You understand the effort that you put into actions and attitudes that others may not notice. And you know your highest hopes and dreams. Life will probably provide you with plenty of critics. Don't make yourself one of them.

84.

Lose Food Rewards

Every day, you face a myriad of challenges, including challenges related to keeping yourself fit and at a healthful weight. One of the ways that many people keep up the good work of meeting life's challenges is to promise themselves rewards. If it works for you, this is a perfectly good strategy. However, for the most part, you will get yourself in trouble if your reward system requires consumption of some sort.

Some people turn to shopping and end up in debt because they spend more on their rewards than they earn from their job well done. Others turn to alcohol, which carries its own obvious and well-known risks. Still others look to food.

If you want to keep your weight within a healthy range, food is probably not the reward of choice. Part of the psychological value of a reward system is that it allows you to focus while you're accomplishing something that would otherwise seem arduous. One of best antidotes to overeating is learning how *not* to make food your focus. Obviously, if you're using food as your reward, you're subverting one of your basic strategies for keeping your weight where you want it.

You don't need to consume in order to reward yourself for your good efforts and accomplished missions. Life is full of pleasures that come free of charge or consequences. A personal day off from time to time can be the greatest gift that you can give to yourself. A great book that you take a whole day to read without interruption can be a luxury that you won't enjoy without making it a priority. Time with a favored friend or family member is more precious than any acquisition, as is a special date with your romantic interest or life partner.

Personal enrichment can also serve as a meaningful reward. When the challenge that you've met has required sustained effort, you may pat yourself on the back with a day-long or semester-long course that teaches you a new skill or hobby, or explores an area of intellectual interest. Many universities and colleges offer courses specifically for adults. Communities also often offer adult opportunities for learning, sports, or fitness. Giving yourself the time to plan a garden or a project can offer great rewards that last a long time.

Your reward options are limited only by your imagination. Don't limit yourself to consumption. Life is too short, and offers too much of value to let consumer goods or food products be your only choices.

85.

Take Control in Restaurants

By now, it should be no mystery that you have choices that can allow you the pleasure of dining out while also keeping you on a balanced track with your weight control. If you have any qualms, just review with yourself the fact that you are the customer. You pay for that meal. There's no reason why you can't ask for what you want, within the ability and policy of the restaurant to provide it. Most restaurateurs these days expect some special requests and honor them.

If you like to dine out, you should probably make sure before you go to a particular eatery that you can ask for minor substitutions or alterations to what is offered. Or see whether they offer meals that are on the light side, either in content or portion size. If you go to a restaurant that tells you straight out that substitutions are not allowed, you can hardly complain when they stick to their policy. It's up to you to find a place that is better suited to your needs and preferences.

Some people lighten the load of a meal by choosing a couple of appetizers as their meal—often a salad plus one of the cooked "starters." Many restaurants have great salad offerings for just a little more than a standard house salad, as well as a choice of good soups and small servings of hot food. This can make a very satisfying meal for someone who has developed the habit of eating raw vegetables and keeping the main dish moderate.

If you're concerned about the fat content of food, ask your server if the restaurant offers any dishes made especially with heart health in mind. Many chefs have developed a short list of dishes that have no cholesterol and a reduced amount of salt in them. Be aware, however, that the chef often chooses to add extra sugar to help enhance the appeal of the food.

It's okay, if everyone at your table agrees, to tell the server not to bother with the breadbasket. If your meal includes pasta, potatoes, or some other starch, you can ask for a small portion of that, substitute a vegetable, or just ask that it stay in the kitchen.

One of the best ways to control what you eat in a restaurant is to ask for all additives—oil, dressing, butter, sour cream, or sauces—on the side. Some of the sauces are actually used in the preparation and can't be put on the side. In that case, ask that the chef use a light hand for your serving. A taste of any of those items can add the flavor that you enjoy at a much-reduced level of intake.

86.

Learn New Measures of Success

Human beings are social animals. We are psychologically designed to live in communities. This presents a challenge, however, because at the same time that we enjoy and even need the company of others, we also tend to compare ourselves with them. We compare where we live, how much money we make, and how we look. If we don't "measure up," we feel like failures, and our self-esteem takes a beating.

This carries over into our struggles with weight. It's not enough that we aren't satisfied with the way that extra weight affects our health and our activities. We don't like the way that it makes us look, and most of the time, we don't like the way we look in comparison to other, trimmer people. The dimension of our bodies has moved up the charts to be one of the major measures we use when we judge success.

A human being's worth does not ultimately reside in externals such as wealth or appearance. A person has intrinsic value without doing, accumulating, or controlling anything. Life itself creates worth. Success does not reside in externals, either. It resides in the qualities of a person's character and actions. Murderous, cruel, and greedy people have made themselves "successes" by measures of personal appearance and wealth. If that's success, we should take failure any day.

Don't fall into the trap of allowing your struggle with weight control to become your personal gauge of success. It can happen subtly. The longer you struggle, the more apt you are to think of yourself as a failure. You may not yet have done what you set out to do, it's true—but it's also true that as long as you're alive, positive change remains possible, and you can continue to take responsibility and try. Success isn't a destination; it's a process that has to do with perseverance and diligence. You only fail if you give up.

87.

Understand the Mechanics of Hunger

Hunger is a gift. Like pain, it tells us something that we need to know if we're going to survive. People who lose the ability to feel pain are in grave danger. The same goes for hunger. Hunger is your body's signal to you that you need nourishment and fuel. If you never felt hungry, and consequently didn't bother to eat, you would starve to death.

There are times, however, when we meet our daily calorie requirements—that is, we take in enough fuel—yet we continue to feel hungry. That's when we have to think again about the quality of how and what we eat. Apparently, hunger sensations are not strictly a matter of keeping the intake at a certain level. Our bodies are more discerning than that. If a lot of the calories that we ingest come from food of questionable nutritional value, our bodies are still in need of adequate nourishment and demand more ingestion.

If you want to offset the feeling of hunger in the midst of limiting your food intake, make very sure that everything you eat has real nutritional value. Remember that a healthful diet includes plenty of fiber. The fiber in a diet actually helps to promote the feeling of being full—not hungry. A sound diet also includes a lot of water, another great aid to not feeling hungry. A good balance of protein, carbohydrates, minerals, vitamins, and fats in several well-apportioned meals a day should leave you satisfied.

It may be that if you continue to feel hungry after you've eaten an adequate amount that you're simply eating too fast. If you eat your meal without taking the time to completely chew, you forestall the first important part of digestion. Chewing not only masticates the food before you send it to your stomach, it stimulates saliva in your mouth. Saliva acts on the food to begin the breakdown that will allow your body to use the food's nutrients.

There are psychological factors at work, too. There is nourishment for the body and nourishment for the soul. Our hunger is not only for physical sustenance but also for pleasurable, satisfying moments. A hunk of food grabbed on the run and virtually swallowed whole does nothing for the needs of your spirit. Taking the time to set a nice table, prepare and present food so that it is aesthetically appealing, and sit with enough time to eat it at leisure will make a difference. Your body will have time to register how much you have eaten before you eat too much, and your senses will have the opportunity to revel in the satisfaction of hunger.

88.

Put Diets in Perspective

When you think "diet," you may automatically think of being "on a diet." Being on a diet carries a load of unpleasant associations: eating food you don't care for; always feeling hungry; having to deprive yourself of the foods you most enjoy. Rather than fall for the modern, product-oriented definition of diet, return to its original meaning—your way of eating. Whatever you typically eat is your diet. You don't have to go on a diet. You already have one. You only have to redesign it so that it better serves your physical needs and personal goals.

This may sound like a game of semantics, but it's not. The "diet" language can become a psychological trap that makes you feel deprived and depressed. It's a short step from there to preoccupation, as though the only important facet of your life is what you eat.

When you think "diet," just think of it as the catch-all term that applies to the types of food you have chosen to make a regular part of your food intake. Then get on with the rest of your life.

89.

Beat the Nibbles in Food Preparation

If you're often or always the one who does the cooking in your household, you've probably noticed how easy it is to nibble as you work. Nibbling can erode a weight-management plan in a hurry, primarily because it's a situation in which you eat almost without being aware that you're doing it. Because you're actually doing something else—cooking—you may not even pay attention to the fact that you're putting food in your mouth. That's a sure recipe for overeating.

If you want to avoid the nibbles altogether, you may find it helpful to always chew gum when you're working in the kitchen. If that's a habit that doesn't appeal, you might try brushing your teeth before you start cooking. Many people find that the fresh flavor in their mouth makes them less interested in eating. It may also, by association, signal the time to *stop* eating.

It may help, as well, to have a big glass of water or a cup of tea on hand. When the urge to put something in your mouth strikes,

186

you can reach for the glass or the cup instead of the food. The beverage has the added advantage of helping you to feel full.

Alternatively, you may want to prepare a planned snack to keep separate from the food that you are preparing. Food that needs chewing, such as vegetable sticks, can give you the oral fix that you want while keeping the calories down and nibbles at bay. A planned snack gives you a measured amount with a beginning and an end. You'll know that you're finished when your snack plate is empty. If you still feel like nibbling, resort to beverages.

The aim here is to know what you are eating and make it a happy fit with what you hope to accomplish. You don't have to give up the pleasure of preparing wonderful meals because the nibbles have been a problem in the past. Create a new present and future.

90.

Help Someone Else

A fine line exists between self-improvement and self-involvement. As with any effort to take responsibility for our lives and well-being, when we put our energy into weight control and fitness, it's easy to pay more attention to our own concerns than those around us. If this imbalance isn't corrected over time, our world becomes a smaller place. Our own troubles and challenges loom large, because we wrap ourselves in them to the neglect of others.

There's no better time than in the midst of self-improvement to reach out to someone else. Instead of focusing all of your energy inward, make up your mind to really listen to those around you. Ask the polite question at the start of a conversation, "How are you?" Then pay attention to the answer, and respond with interest and sympathy. Call a friend you haven't seen for a while, just to check in and say that you're thinking of him or her. Be in touch with family, and make *them* the center of attention for a while.

You may know someone who, like you, wants to get his or her

weight under control. This could be an opportunity to be a support to someone else in an arena whose struggles you know well. It's one of the ways that the challenges in life can be transformed into something good and valuable. When you can say with meaning and sympathy, "I know what you're talking about, and I'm with you," you offer a gift of great value.

Other people's lives don't stop when your own becomes preoccupying. Others face daily problems and frustrations, too. They need as much support as you do. You can be part of their support, even when you need it in return. Mutual concern is at the heart of community. When you play your part, your world expands, and you can more readily put your personal concerns in perspective.

91.

Balance Appearance with Effect

As you get to know a person better, it's inevitable that your first impression will be affected by what you know about his or her personality and character. Their actions speak, as does their attitude toward others. If you find them attractive as people, you will almost certainly find them physically attractive, too. That's true in reverse, as well. The better people get to know *you*, the more they will focus on the person you are and put your physical appearance in that context.

When you're working on weight loss and management, you may find yourself focusing on external qualities. Zero in on that tendency, and resist it. What and who you are as a person is what will last, long after age has done its work on your looks.

Obviously, this isn't to say that you should forget about weight control. It is to say that your appearance is only part of the picture. The more you keep that in mind and give equal or better attention to grooming your character and temperament, the batter balanced your life with yourself and others will be.

92.

Chart Your Progress

When you launch a weight-loss effort, the road ahead can look long and difficult. Setting short-range goals can make the effort less daunting, as can charting the progress that you make.

All you need is a simple notebook or calendar. You may want to include a graph paper chart of some kind so that you can actually create a picture of your progress. Keep it somewhere that you feel free to be honest. If you think other people will see it, you may be tempted to cheat, so make it your business alone.

Record your starting weight, and if you want, your dimensions— chest, waist, and hips. Decide how often you can weigh in without it becoming a preoccupation. At whatever interval you choose (once a week is best), record your latest weight. If you weigh yourself at about the same time of day with approximately the same amount of clothing on, you'll get the most accurate reading. When you're charting progress, it's less important what the specific numbers are than what they are in relation to your last weight.

Between weigh-ins, create a daily space for recording physical activity. Exercise is a vital part of healthy weight control, and it can be motivating to see how often you fulfill your intention to be active. Some people find a regular dose of the same exercise the easiest to sustain. Others like to "cross-train"—that is, to have several different types of exercise that they do in rotation. What you choose is less important than that you get regular exercise. The best exercise routine is worthless if you can't sustain it.

Once a month, at most, measure your dimensions again. If you're faithfully active in exercising while you lose weight, you will begin to see the numbers change. In fact, that may be where you see the most progress. Muscle really does weigh more than fat, so as you become more fit, your weight may change less than you expected, while you still show remarkable results in your appearance.

We all have our moments of discouragement. A chart of your progress can remind you that you are doing the hard work that results in positive change.

93.

Never Finish Your Food

You add untold calories to your daily intake when you let the size of a portion on your plate dictate how much you eat. You may have little or no control over portion size in some situations, but you can always control how much of that portion you decide to put in your mouth.

Habits tend to become unconscious actions. That's why we call them habits. We repeat them so often that they become default behavior. If you have developed the habit of finishing every bite, it's time to start thinking at the table again. Conscious action is one of your best defenses against unneeded consumption. Eat slowly. Put your fork down after each bite. Let your appestat—your internal hunger gauge—have time to register how much you've eaten. When you no longer feel hungry, *stop eating*. Never mind how much food is still sitting on your plate. Remember: When it comes to food that has already been served to you, it's a choice of waste or waist.

For the die-hard plate cleaner, more aggressive action may be needed. Some people have found it helpful to create a new habit of *never* finishing the food on their plates. It can be as little as a single bite, but if you make up your mind to leave at least that much, you'll grow more comfortable with pushing the plate away before you've polished it off. You'll also send the signal to whomever's serving you that you've had enough and would prefer to do without the seconds. It's much more convincing to say, "No, thanks, I've had enough," when you don't scrape up the last tiny morsel.

94.

Develop Healthful Food Relationships

Food is a necessity. It is, happily, also a pleasure. But when weight loss becomes the central factor in a person's relationship with food, it can come to look like the enemy. What a shame.

Don't let your concerns for a healthy weight rob you of a healthy appreciation of food, both for its nutritional value and the sensual satisfaction that it can give. Your body operates as a complex system of various smaller systems that interact and balance constantly. Circulatory, nervous, digestive, and endocrine systems each play their parts in keeping the entire organism working and well. Food and water are its fuel—but your attitude plays its part.

The way that you think and feel has a documented effect on how your body functions. You have probably experienced this when you have been unhappy, angry, or upset, and your digestive system registers your emotions in loss of appetite, nausea, or stomach pains. Your feelings and attitudes can also affect your breathing, blood pressure, and hormones. Negative attitudes about food may actually change the way that you are able to digest and metabolize the food that you eat.

Don't think of food as your adversary. It is just food—sustenance, potential energy, and possible pleasure. When you cook for yourself or order food in a restaurant, take the time to be grateful that you have enough to eat, and that the food available to you is wholesome and plentiful. It plays a crucial role in your life, but it is just one small part of a complicated whole. You consist of more than what you ingest. You can appreciate it without overeating or fixating.

95.

Resist Madison Avenue

An enormous amount of corporate money is funneled into advertising, which makes it exciting and monetarily rewarding for those who have the ability for it. For the rest of us, this means that not only do endless sales pitches surround us, but those messages are designed and conveyed in highly sophisticated and appealing ways that can grab and convince us without our even being aware of it.

For the next week, pay conscious attention to how many advertisements you are exposed to that have to do with food, diets, fitness, weight loss, or exercise. Add the predominant images in other sorts of advertising—slim, beautiful people having happy, sexy, successful encounters over food and drinks; or the same slim, beautiful people exercising with the precision and strength of professional athletes or dancers.

The messages are constant and affecting. They are also sometimes subtle, and we hardly realize that we are taking them in and making them a part of our view of others and ourselves. But our self-image suffers. Our definition of "slim and beautiful" takes on the coloration of the professional models that we see in the ads. Our desire to look like them and live the fictional lives that they portray attaches itself to a long list of products. We become consumers of the message, as much as we do of the goods and services that the message is meant to sell.

Given our media-driven culture, resisting the influence of advertising can be a challenging task at best. It requires that we notice when we're being offered images and ideas designed to sell something. It also demands that we take the messages apart and grow to understand the secondary messages that affect the way that we see ourselves.

The more you notice, the better you'll be at putting the ads in their place and refusing their power over your attitudes and perceptions. You may even decide to reconsider some of the publications that you buy and programs that you watch, because the advertising they use does not help you keep moving forward. Be aware and take the time to know what is truly important to you. The advertising images are a poor substitute for your real life.

96.

Balance Appetite with Attitude

Appetite—the desire to eat—is a great boon to good health and should be seen as such. But it has its tricky aspects, and you'll do well to be aware of those, too. A physical need for sustenance can drive your appetite. But so can many other influences: a beautiful picture of a well-presented goodie of some sort; the sight of someone else eating something that you find appetizing; a social event that offers food at a time when you don't need or want to eat; or simply the resolution not to eat some particular item.

When you decide to take control of your weight and your eating habits, you can help your efforts considerably by thinking through, in specific terms, why you're doing it, what you hope for in the long run, and how much it matters to you. This thought process will allow you to develop positive attitudes about your efforts. These become your tools when appetite strikes.

When you feel like eating, stop and determine why. Then let your attitudes about managing weight act as a counterbalance to the desire to eat. The point is not to say no every time that appetite hits, but rather to know why you make the decision to eat or not. Just going through the conscious process will help you to form new habits that keep you moving in the direction that you want to go. In fact, the thought process itself can become a valuable habit that can serve you in other areas, as well.

The bottom line is this: Appetite comes from your mind, as well as your body. Use your head, and you'll be able to keep appetite in its place.

97.

Feature Seasonal Foods in Your Diet

Before people had refrigeration, they focused on eating what was available locally, in season, or what could be preserved. With the advent of refrigeration and high-speed transportation, we have entered an age in which we can find virtually any food from almost anyplace in the world right in our hometowns. This adds a great deal to the variety and interest in our daily diets. But it may not always serve our best interests for weight management.

For long-term success, weight management depends on your ability to feel satisfied when you've eaten enough for good health. Food that has been grown and marketed locally is almost always fresher than shipped food, which means that it retains more of its natural nutrients, flavor, and texture. Because it offers more intrinsic value and aesthetic appeal, it has the potential to be more satisfying than food that has been refrigerated, stored, and shipped.

Local food also offers a natural way to keep your meals interesting without a lot of added fat and sugar. The available produce, especially, changes regularly, as various items reach their peak, and then peter out. Because the food is at its best in flavor, it needs little or no enhancement. It tends to suit the season in which it grows—sweet, watery fruits and leafy vegetables in spring and summer; storable, sustaining fruits and higher-carbohydrate vegetables as the weather gets colder—making it all the more enjoyable.

Get to know what local farmers produce in your area. Find out where they sell their products, and make it a point to frequent those places. Enjoy plenty of the fresh fruits and vegetables that you can eat raw. They are a wonderful source of nutrients, fiber, and water, and are almost universally low in calories and free of fat.

You can make seasonal food the centerpiece of your meals because it is fresh, delicious, and nice to look at. Let the heavier foods—refined starches and meats—take a backseat for a change. You'll have a ready way to keep your meals interesting and light.

98.

Know the Symptoms of Eating Disorders

The study of the eating disorders, anorexia nervosa and bulimia, has become part of the health curriculum for students in middle and high school. They figure prominently in many mental health practices. And they are the subjects of much research and clinical study. All of this activity reflects the fact that these diseases are almost commonplace today, and no one should remain ignorant of either their symptoms or their dangers. It has been shown that people who engage in drastic dieting or extreme exercising are more apt to develop eating disorders than people whose food and body-related behaviors are more moderate.

Bulimia is characterized by frequent binge eating followed by purging. Anorexia is distinguished by self-starvation. Both diseases show up in male and female populations, and among children, young adults, and adults. They are notoriously difficult to remedy, and they are life-threatening.

If you are a perennial dieter in search of the next quick-loss plan, or if you are a fanatical exerciser, you need to pay attention to the dangers of eating disorders. A diet that calls for massive amounts of a single food creates an imbalance in your eating habits that can snowball into disordered eating. So, too, can an overemphasis on body shape and size. Much helpful material is available from health professionals, and a number of fine books have been published on the subject. Check out a book from your local library, and understand what eating disorders are all about. If nothing else, the information will offer a poignant reminder of how lopsided and destructive a preoccupation with weight can become.

99.

Rethink the Treats in Your Kitchen

Even when you're working on weight loss and management, there's room for the occasional treat. But as we all know, treats can quickly get out of control. As with other aspects of weight control, you do yourself a big favor when you take steps to give yourself the best shot at success.

First, rethink the *kinds* of food that you treat yourself to. Avoid empty-calorie treats. Instead, think about goodies that include some nutritive value—nuts, grains, fruit, or seeds. Trail mix usually makes for a better choice than fatty chips, for example. If you must have a piece of chocolate, make it one of the nut-filled kinds, so that you're at least getting a little protein. Consider having a whole-grain muffin instead of a sweet roll. If you have a yen for a sweet, try dried fruit rather than hard candy. The idea is to make sure that you get some food value. If the goodies in your kitchen are all wholesome, nutritious foods, you'll have an easier time avoiding the junk foods.

Second, remember that *quantity* counts. Even the most nutritious, weight-conscious choices will subvert your goals if you eat too much of them. When you buy treats for home, buy them in small quantities. Many foods are available in pint-size packages, as well as giant, economy sizes. Go for small. It will make it more difficult to keep eating when it's time to stop. If the foods that you choose only come in quantity, divide them up into single-serving packages as soon as you bring them home. With a prepackaged amount, you have a built-in stopping point for your treat time.

Third, think carefully about *where* you store your goodies. If you choose refrigerator food, put the treats out of sight on a lower shelf, behind the salad fixings. Or store your treats in a hard-to-reach cupboard that you don't often need to visit. If your treat food is hard to reach or well hidden, you're more likely to forget about it or decide that it's too much trouble.

Finally, remember *why* you've chosen to have the occasional treat. Maybe your energy drops off now and then, and a treat gives you a lift. Or perhaps you've discovered that your attitude toward a healthful diet improves when you give yourself that once-in-a-while change. Consciously remembering the reasons for treating yourself in the context of your long-range goal of weight management can offer just the right brake mechanism to keep you from overindulging.

100.

Get Over It

So you've decided that you're going to get your weight under control and keep it that way. You've established short- and long-range goals for positive changes in your lifestyle. You're taking charge of what you eat, and you're making a point of including more physical activity in your daily routine. That's great.

There's just one more move to make, and that's to keep it up for long enough and with enough consistency that it genuinely becomes your new norm. The automatic nature of habit is both its bane and beauty. It can hold you back when you want to make positive changes, but it can also allow you to establish new ways of eating and exercising that help you reach your goals for good.

The best part of making healthy eating and exercising a habit is that you can end your preoccupation with it. It doesn't have to be the centerpiece of your life anymore. You can let go of the endless glances in the mirror and get on with living. You can establish a new view of your body and your strength of purpose, and then forget to think about it.

Habits can be made or broken in about six weeks. Six weeks, in the context of a lifetime, is a short time indeed. Apply yourself to just six weeks of conscious, constant attention to the habits that will serve you for a lifetime. Then let the habits prevail, and get over the fixation with weight. Life itself is the best sweet offering.